Postgraduate Medical Education and training

A guide for primary and secondary care

Edited by

Anne Hastie
Director of Postgraduate General Practice, London Deanery

Ian Hastie
Dean of Postgraduate Medicine, London Deanery
Consultant and Senior Lecturer
St George's Hospital and Medical School, London

Neil Jackson
Dean of Postgraduate General Practice Education, London Deanery
Honorary Professor of Medical Education
Barts and the London Hospitals

Forewords by
Professor Sir Graeme Catto
Professor Elisabeth Paice

Radcliffe Publishing
Oxford • Seattle

Radcliffe Publishing Ltd
18 Marcham Road
Abingdon
Oxon OX14 1AA
United Kingdom

www.radcliffe-oxford.com
Electronic catalogue and worldwide online ordering facility.

British Library Cataloguing in Publication Data

A catalogue record for this book is available from the British Library.

ISBN 1 85775 628 2

Typeset by Ann Buchan (Typesetters), Shepperton, Middlesex
Printed and bound by T J International Ltd, Padstow, Cornwall

Contents

Foreword

We are living through upheaval in postgraduate medical education and training, but not before time.

The content of training is being recast through the *Modernising Medical Careers* initiatives. At first the main focus was on the new Foundation Programme and streamlining specialist and GP training. From the start, however, *Modernising Medical Careers* was intended also to address the needs and aspirations of those outside the NHS training grades.

At the same time, the Postgraduate Medical Education and Training Board has been set up to modernise the institutional relationships, to bring coherence and consistency to standard setting and quality assurance, to prepare for the new GP Register and to establish new ways on to the Specialist Register. Postgraduate education and training remains crowded with organisations, however, and the Board is legally obliged to co-operate with the Royal Colleges and with the GMC in particular.

The GMC is also obliged to co-operate with its partners. Like the Board, we would not want it any other way and indeed could achieve little in glorious isolation. The GMC's Education Committee also has the legal function of 'co-ordinating all stages of medical education'. The Committee therefore includes members of the GMC alongside nominees from bodies involved in undergraduate and postgraduate education and training.

The goal of the co-ordination is to achieve a continuum in medical education, from entry to medical school to retirement from medical practice. Students and doctors can demonstrate their professional development through outcomes-based education and training and formative and summative assessment. As they specialise, they must not lose the generic attributes set out by the GMC in *Good Medical Practice*. Postgraduate training and education cannot be only about technical skills if patients are to come first and doctors are to remain fit to practise.

The Education Committee of the GMC has been putting five questions to the providers of medical education and training. How do we prepare students and doctors for patient-centred care? What do we mean by learner-centred education and training? Are we doing enough to promote equality and value diversity? How can we contribute to the development of inter-professional learning and practice? And how on earth can we prepare today's students and doctors for decades of progress in medical possibilities and patients' expectations?

There is a full agenda, then. We can be forgiven if at times we find the pace of change a little confusing or even alarming. But the potential for good is enormous. The contributions in this book report progress so far and indicate the extent of the commitment and talent to hand. Through co-operation and co-ordination, we can build on this investment and the potential for good can be achieved.

Professor Sir Graeme Catto
President
General Medical Council
January 2005

Foreword

Postgraduate medical education is something that the UK is widely recognised as being good at. Doctors from all over the world are attracted to the opportunity to train in a variety of specialties and settings under educational and clinical supervision. One of the unique features of the UK system in the last decade has been the developing role of the Postgraduate Deanery. The Deanery is responsible for making sure that each training programme offers the range of experience and the degree of supervision required and has a supportive educational framework in place. The Deanery ensures that each trainee is selected fairly and transparently; is given an informative induction to each placement; has clear educational objectives and a personal development plan; has the chance to learn through doing, under supervision; is regularly appraised and assessed; and if his or her performance is a concern, is informed of this and supported in dealing with the problem. A tall order.

This book describes the history of postgraduate medical education in the UK, and how the role of the Postgraduate Deanery developed and changed to suit the needs of an NHS that is chronically short of doctors, and where the tension between service and training has sometimes seemed about to reach breaking point. It sets postgraduate medical education in the context of change in the NHS, with a massive agenda for modernisation affecting every aspect of primary and secondary care. It reviews the roles of the various organisations that are involved in the standard setting, quality assurance and provision of postgraduate education. Refreshingly, the editors have wherever possible ensured that the issues for primary and secondary care are dealt with together, discouraging tribalism and encouraging the spread of good practice. It tackles issues such as human rights and equal opportunities legislation as they apply to training, e-learning, management of poor performance and life-long learning. The authors are drawn from staff working in or closely with the London Deanery, who deal with the issues they describe on a daily basis, and who speak from their experience. Here is a guide of interest and practical use to all those engaged in the management or delivery of postgraduate medical education.

Professor Elisabeth Paice
Dean Director
London Deanery
January 2005

About the editors

Anne Hastie

Director of Postgraduate General Practice, London Deanery. A full-time general practitioner in South London for 25 years before joining the London Deanery. During her time in general practice, Dr Hastie was a GP trainer, GP tutor and Adviser for Non-Principal GPs. She has a special interest in flexible training and working, GP returners and prolonged study leave. In 2000 she received an MBE for services to primary care.

Ian Hastie

Dean of Postgraduate Medicine, London Deanery, and Consultant and Senior Lecturer at St George's Hospital and Medical School, London. President of the Geriatric Medicine Section of the European Union Medical Specialties, a member of the Specialist Advisory Committee for Geriatric Medicine and member of the National Training Committee of the British Geriatrics Society.

Neil Jackson

Professor Neil Jackson first entered general practice in 1974 (he retired from active clinical practice in 1999 after 25 years as a full-time principal) and quickly developed an interest in education and training. He is a former GP trainer, course organiser and associate regional adviser in general practice. He is now Postgraduate Dean for General Practice in the London Deanery and Honorary Professor of Medical Education at Barts and the London hospitals. He is a former MRCGP Examiner and the author of various books, book chapters, peer-referenced papers and articles on general practice/primary care/education and training issues. For the past several years he has worked as Visiting Primary Care Consultant in countries of the former Russian Federation, including Georgia and Uzbekistan and more recently in Japan.

List of contributors

Tareq Abouharb

GP principal since 1997 at the Limes Medical Centre in Epping, Essex, and Task Orientated Associate Director for the Higher Professional Education (HPE) programme at the London Deanery since 2001. Helped to establish a team of programme directors responsible for the running of HPE in the deanery's five sectors. Present areas of focus: developing the HPE programme content, modes of delivery and access; working with Deanery colleagues to further support GPs at key times of transition in their professional lives; representing the London Deanery on the national evaluation team for HPE.

Antony Americano

Antony Americano is currently Head of Human Resources and Central Services at the London Department of Postgraduate Medical and Dental Education, University of London. He is a Fellow of the Chartered Institute of Personnel and Development and has a Masters degree in Organisational Behaviour from Birkbeck College, University of London.

Jane Appleyard

Medical Workforce Project Manager, London Deanery. Read Mediaeval and Modern History at Nottingham University before joining the House of Fraser as a management trainee. Worked in Medical Personnel as a locum at Central Middlesex Hospital, ending up at the Deanery after posts at The Middlesex Hospital, Bloomsbury Health Authority and St George's Hospital. Member of the Chartered Institute of Personnel and Development.

Rhamesh Bhatt

Associate Director, Department of Postgraduate General Practice Education. Patch Associate Director for West London where he lives and works as a general practitioner. Professional Executive Committee member of Ealing Primary Care Trust in West London.

Graeme Catto

Professor Sir Graeme Catto is President of the General Medical Council, Vice-Principal at King's College London, Dean of the Guy's, King's College and St Thomas' Hospitals' Medical and Dental School and Pro-Vice Chancellor, University of London. After graduating in medicine, he obtained a Harkness

Fellowship to study at Harvard University. He is an honorary physician with an interest in renal medicine and has published widely on different aspects of nephrology and immunology. Formerly Chief Scientist at the Scottish Executive Health Department, he is currently a member of South East London Strategic Health Authority and the Council for Healthcare Regulatory Excellence.

Nav Chana

General practitioner in Mitcham, Surrey, Associate Director London Deanery, RCGP examiner and Co-chair RCGP Workplace Assessment Development Group.

Robert Clarke

Bob Clarke is Associate Director of Postgraduate General Practice in the London Deanery. His educational interests are in the role of reflection in learning, interprofessional learning and communication skills training. He is co-author of a book, *Critical Reading for the Reflective Practitioner* (Butterworth Heinemann, 1998) and has recently joined a clinical skills website (www.askdoctorclarke.com). He is a Fellow of the Royal College of General Practitioners and of the Royal College of Physicians, and is a member of the Higher Education Academy.

Ian Curran

Clinical Tutor and Assistant Director Bart's Medical Simulation Centre, Consultant Anaesthetist and Pain Management Specialist, St Bartholomew's and The Royal London Hospitals. Interested in the delivery of novel postgraduate training within the hospital context. The training of professional, non-technical skills must be a core NHS activity if patient care is to improve. Developing practitioner insight into the many areas of professional competence such as crisis management, mentoring, teamworking, conflict negotiation and consultation skills is often challenging and highly rewarding. His interest in the complex world of professional meta-competencies stems largely from his own clinical and training needs.

Caroline Doherty

Mentoring programme co-ordinator with the Education Support Unit, a London Deanery initiative. In this role Caroline developed mentoring programmes for doctors and nurses in London (with GPs in north-west London, with GPs and nurses at Haringey Teaching Primary Care Trust and with new consultants in a number of trusts). A learning and professional development specialist whose professional background includes vocational counselling, training management, social work and postgraduate medical education. Now works independently and offers consultancy to mentoring programme organisers, develops and supports mentors, and evaluates mentoring programmes.

Charles Easmon

Professor Easmon holds a chair at Thames Valley University where, following his retirement from the Department of Health in 2003, he was invited to establish a centre for the study of policy and practice in health and social care.

He is also Deputy Chairman of the Health Protection Agency, an Associate Non-Executive Director of the South West London Health Authority and Chair of its Workforce Development Board and a visiting professor at Imperial College. A microbiologist by training, Professor Easmon became Dean of Postgraduate Medicine in the University of London in 1992, and from 1994 was Director of Education and Training and then Workforce Development, first for the North Thames Region and then for the London Region of the National Health Service.

Beverley Gainey
Head of Educational Resource Development, BA (Hons) MBA (Cranfield) CPFA; worked for ICI, Inland Revenue, National Audit Office, National Health Service, Department of Health and the London Deanery.

Imtiaz Gulamali
Has a broad range of experience in both primary and secondary care as well as in general practice education. Worked as a hospital practitioner and also Lead for Diabetes in a primary care trust. Worked as a GP tutor for five years and at present is trainer, course organiser and Associate Director in the London Deanery.

Owen Hanmer
Associate Dean for Specialties at the London Deanery since 2001, also a consultant paediatrician at the Royal London Hospital and Tower Hamlets Primary Care Trust. Previously held posts in postgraduate medical education as a clinical tutor, college regional adviser and speciality training committee chair, and in clinical management as a clinical director and medical director. Actively involved in the development of assessment and appraisal in the Royal College of Paediatrics and Child Health, and in the London Deanery in developing competence-based recruitment processes for specialist registrars, help for doctors in difficulty, training for trainers and mentoring for trainees.

Shelley Heard
Deputy Dean Director, London Deanery. Trained as a medical microbiologist at St Bartholomew's Hospital Medical School. As a Senior Lecturer/Honorary Consultant at St Bartholomew's and the Homerton, in Microbiology, she developed managerial and educational interests which resulted in her being appointed Chief Executive of the Homerton Hospital in the east end of London. Subsequently became Dean of Postgraduate Medicine, initially for North Central London, and then subsequently for the London Deanery. She has particular interests in workforce issues, academic developments and e-learning.

John Krapez
Consultant Anaesthetist and Clinical Tutor at Barts and The London NHS Trust. Involved with training and education since the mid-1970s, initially with undergraduates and subsequently with postgraduate and continuing medical education. Given charge of introducing the Calman training reforms to the

second biggest trust in the UK, he realised early on the importance of educating the trainers (both present and future) and has been involved in developing a number of courses aimed at providing the skills and knowledge needed by this vital group of doctors.

Anthea Lints
Director of Postgraduate Education in the London Deanery and a part-time principle in a practice in Chelmsford, Essex. Deanery responsibilities include recruitment and career advice.

Yong-Lock Ong
Associate Dean, Overseas Office, London Deanery, Consultant Psychiatrist, Psychiatry of Old Age, North East London Mental Health Trust, Goodmayes Hospital, Essex IG3 8YB.

Victor Orton
Head of Medical Workforce at the London Deanery. Responsible for the recruitment of specialist registrars, their annual assessments and administrative support to the specialty training committees. Involved with doctors in difficulty and litigation. Worked in the National Health Service and with associated employers in London since July 1973, specialising in human resources roles.

Elisabeth Paice
Professor Elisabeth Paice is Dean Director of Postgraduate Medical and Dental Education for London (2001–present). She was previously Consultant Rheumatologist at Whittington Hospital, where she was also Clinical Tutor (1990–1993). She became Associate Dean for North East Thames in 1993 with special responsibility for pre-registration house officers, senior house officers and flexible training. In 1995 she became Dean Director of Postgraduate Medical and Dental Education for North Thames. She has published on medical careers, the impact of recent reforms to postgraduate medical training, factors causing stress and disillusionment in trainee doctors, aspects of the relationship between trainers and trainees, and appraisal and the management of performance in trainees.

Timothy Peters
Timothy Peters retired in 2004. He was Professor of Clinical Biochemistry and Sub-dean for Higher Degrees and Postgraduate Degrees at the School of Medicine at King's College, University of London. He was seconded part-time to the London Department of Postgraduate Medical and Dental Education (LPMDE) for a number of years prior to his retirement. At LPMDE he was closely involved in promoting Flexible Training in Postgraduate Medical Education.

Wendy Reid
Postgraduate Dean in London and a consultant gynaecologist at the Royal Free Hospital, London.

Suzanne Savage
GP in South London for 29 years and has been a trainer for most of that time. She was a course organiser for the Guy's and St Thomas' GP vocational training scheme for 10 years before becoming Associate Dean for South East London, a post she has held for the last 10 years.

John Spicer
GP in Croydon for nearly 20 years. Associate Director of GP Education for the south-east sector of the London Deanery and Clinical Tutor in Medical Law and Ethics at St George's Hospital Medical School, London.

Colin Stern
Consultant Paediatrician at Guy's and St Thomas' hospitals since 1980. Visiting Professor, King Saud University, 1986–1987. Clinical Director of Paediatrics 1989–1992. Student Adviser 1984–2003. Responsible for PRHO appointments from 1981 to 1997. Postgraduate Sub-Dean UMDS, later GKT Medical School, 1989–1997. Associate Postgraduate Dean, South Thames Deanery from January 2000 to March 2001. Associate Postgraduate Dean, London Deanery since April 2001, responsible for south-east London, three medical specialities and for career counselling for London trainees. Past President, Paediatric Section and Chairman, Academic Board, Royal Society of Medicine from 2003 to the present date.

Penny Trafford
Associate Director in the London Deanery and working part-time as a GP in north London. Lead for Overseas Doctors Unit in Postgraduate Department of General Practice. Projects being undertaken for the Deanery include induction for overseas doctors, clinical experience scheme for refugee and overseas doctors, setting up protected GP training schemes for refugee doctors and the EU GP Induction Programme.

Alex Trompetas
Associate Director in a primary care development unit dealing with GP performance issues. Lead for Fresh Start remedial programmes in London. Practising GP in a large training practice in south London and also GP Adviser to South East London Strategic Health Authority.

Rebecca Viney
Associate Director of Postgraduate General Practice education for salaried and freelance GPs at the London Deanery. Has been a GP principal, GP retainer, salaried and locum in her time, and is currently a Flexible Career Scheme GP. For the last eight years she has been involved both nationally and via the London Deanery with the education of non-principal GPs. She has organised three national conferences on continuing professional development for GP non-principals, each attracted contributions from all over the UK. The proceedings were published as supplements to the journal *Education for Primary Care*.

Julia Whiteman

Deputy GP Director for the London Deanery. She is a GP with over 20 years experience in general practice as a partner and latterly as a freelance GP. Responsible for the Primary Care Development Unit in the London Deanery, which includes leading on work with GP performance cases.

Introduction

With a huge Government programme of development and modernisation in the National Health Service (NHS) currently in progress comes the need to understand the NHS education and training system, and its role in promoting quality healthcare. Quality in the primary and secondary care sectors of the NHS can only be achieved by a system of service delivery that is supported and informed by the systems of education and training, and research and development, that is, a 'three systems approach'.[1]

The doctors of today, and those in the future, must have appropriate knowledge, skills and attitudes to meet the challenge of a fast-changing world: medical advances, new technologies and new approaches to patient care. In addition to being highly trained and motivated they must also become lifelong learners and reflective practitioners for the duration of their working lives.

This volume sets out to explore the various components of the NHS education and training system, and how it supports doctors in postgraduate training programmes and thereafter in their continuing professional development (CPD). It brings together a group of committed and experienced medical and non-medical professionals, who collectively review the system and give an up-to-date and comprehensive account of its present state and future development.

The editors of the book also seek to facilitate and promote strategic thinking and planning in relation to education and training at various levels, including organisational, team and individual healthcare professionals.

Carter and Jackson[2] have previously described a primary care strategy for education and training, the key elements of which also apply to secondary care. These are as follows.

- NHS organisations need to build in a clear education and training agenda into their developmental programmes, which should include an understanding of workforce planning and multiprofessional or multidisciplinary skill mixes.
- Effective leadership for education and training must be established (in primary and secondary care), which is linked to clinical governance and quality healthcare.
- The various education and training funding streams must be understood in order to ensure that full advantage is taken of all available financial resources.

- Learning and development must occur at various levels in the NHS, whether in the primary or secondary care settings, for example hospital trusts, primary care trusts, general practice and in the community.
- Personal learning and development should be linked to organisational learning and development, for example in general practice, the concept of personal development plans (PDPs) should be linked to practice professional development plans (PPDPs).
- Learning will need to take place across professional and organisational boundaries, for example across the primary and secondary care sectors in the NHS.
- Promoting a greater understanding of the roles of existing educational organisations or structures and their educational networks, for example medical schools and postgraduate departments of medicine or general practice, higher education institutes, etc.
- Developing the concept of 'fitness for purpose' to ensure that a highly skilled and integrated multidisciplinary workforce of healthcare professionals work and learn together to deliver the future NHS agenda for patient care.

Although fitness for practice remains of great importance for doctors and healthcare professionals, fitness for purpose has become increasingly significant in the NHS over the last few years. The concept of fitness for purpose is explored in greater detail in other chapters of this book.

The editors intend that the readers of this book should include healthcare professionals and organisations in the NHS, including strategic health authorities, acute and mental health trusts and primary care trusts, medical and non-medical undergraduate and postgraduate students, patients and lay members of the public.

They also consider that this book could act as a useful reference work to countries outside the UK, some of which are developing healthcare systems based on our own UK model. It is hoped that through its many contributors the book will also provide both theoretical and practical guidance for those delivering and receiving education and training at home or abroad.

The editors would like to acknowledge their particular thanks to Professor Charles Easmon for writing the chapter on the history of deaneries and to Professor Sir Graeme Catto and Professor Elisabeth Paice for writing the Forewords of the book. Thanks go also to the chapter authors, who have contributed so willingly their experience and enthusiasm, without which this book would not have been possible. Lastly, we thank the trainees who are our future.

Anne Hastie
Ian Hastie
Neil Jackson
January 2005

References

1   Jackson N (1999) Quality in the new NHS – the role of education and training in general practice and primary care. *Education for General Practice.* **10**: 6–8.

2   Carter Y and Jackson N (eds) (2002) *Guide to Education and Training for Primary Care.* Oxford University Press, Oxford.

CHAPTER 1

Historial background of deaneries as NHS organisations

Charles Easmon

The profession of medicine

Postgraduate medical education (PGME) and continuing professional development (CPD) together make a rich pie into which many fingers are dipped. In common with the rest of the National Health Service (NHS) the pace of change in medical education is increasing remorselessly. Here, as in other areas, there is some concern that even if the aims of change are laudable, the pace of change is too fast to allow for the time needed for the necessary attitudinal change required for long-term sustainability. The aim of this chapter is to examine the evolving relationship between the NHS and postgraduate medical deaneries. It is important to set this in the broader context of the relationship between the profession of medicine and society, and government at large. The deaneries play a central role, not only in PGME and CPD but also in the management of medical workforce supply. They form a bridge between the Government and the management of the NHS, on the one hand, and the institutions of the medical profession and of higher education, on the other. This will never be an easy position, but it can and should be an influential one, where there is a role for leadership and vision.

The position of the medical profession in the UK developed over the nineteenth century and during the first part of the twentieth century. Medicine became established as a learned profession with a distinct knowledge base, a clear ethical code and standards of behaviour and practice, a tradition of service to patients and the public and of self-regulation. Doctors acquired considerable autonomy and power, and the respect of society. The main medical institutions were:

- The General Medical Council (GMC) (self-regulation, professional standards and education).

- The medical royal colleges (professional standards, education and specialist practice).
- The British Medical Association (BMA) (trade union and professional advocate).
- The medical schools (education and research and development).
- Various learned and professional societies.

The role of the Government was limited, and was most evident in areas such as public health. Within the medical profession there was a clear differentiation in status and power between the hospital-based consultants and general practitioners. The power of the former was based in the royal colleges and in the medical schools and their associated teaching hospitals, whereas the latter looked increasingly to the BMA.

The creation of the NHS

Then, in 1948, the NHS was created, with a virtual monopoly of medical employment: directly in the case of consultants, and indirectly for general practitioners. Central Government funding from general taxation became the prime financial mechanism for delivering healthcare, just at the time when a series of clinical and technological advances greatly increased its scope, complexity and cost. Once the Government became so deeply involved in healthcare it was inevitable that sooner or later it would begin to intervene and manage the process of health service provision, including the closer scrutiny and control of the activities, education and training of the medical profession.

The medical schools and faculties, under the regulation of the GMC, controlled undergraduate medical education and the subsequent period of provisional registration. In the 1950s and early 1960s PGME had a much looser structure. Senior house officers, registrars and senior registrars, working as NHS employees in consultant-led firms, sat the higher diplomas of the royal colleges and acquired the practical experience that would enable them to compete for NHS consultant posts. However, outside the main teaching centres, there was little structured provision of educational facilities and training. PGME stood as much for postgraduate medical *experience* as for *education*. In academic clinical medicine there were research fellowships and lecturer posts. There was even less structure for aspiring general practitioners, although from 1948 a few general practice training posts were established under the supervision of the local medical committees. The third phase of medical education, CPD, was left to the individual as a member of the profession.

A number of recurring themes can be identified:

- conflict between the needs of PGME for trainees, and for service priorities, where trainees are a key part of service delivery

- the merits of the apprentice model against the more academic approach to medical education
- professional autonomy and accountability, and suspicion and resentment of Government attempts to decrease the former and increase the latter
- recurrent crises of medical morale.

From Christchurch to *Working for Patients*

In 1961 the various organisations involved in PGME or CPD, including the Government, came together at the Christchurch Conference to look at its future. This was one of the most significant meetings in the history of postgraduate and continuing medical education. From it came the idea of deans of postgraduate medical education, associated with university medical schools, but with responsibility for overseeing the education and training of 'junior' hospital doctors, largely employed by the NHS. In parallel came local postgraduate medical centres, libraries and other educational facilities, which were developed with the staff necessary to run them. Local consultants were appointed as clinical tutors to head the centres and to act as co-ordinators of medical education, and these networks became part of the postgraduate deans' responsibilities. Although some NHS money went into the centres, much was raised locally. Successful centres established themselves as a focus of medical life, in particular in district general hospitals, attracting not only hospital doctors but also local general practitioners (GPs). For junior hospital staff, the postgraduate medical centre provided one of the few opportunities for them to meet local GPs. The National Association of Clinical Tutors (NACT) was founded in 1969.

In 1971 the first regional advisers in general practice were appointed, and they became responsible, as part of the postgraduate deans' organisations, both for the training of prospective GPs and for the further development of GP principals. GP course organisers took responsibility for PGME, whilst GP tutors became responsible for CPD. Whereas the medical royal colleges set the standards for hospital doctors who wanted to specialise, it was the Joint Committee on Postgraduate Training for General Practitioners (JCPTGP) (founded in 1976) rather than the Royal College of General Practitioners (RCGP), which became responsible for issuing certificates at the end of successful completion of GP training.

During the 1970s, with the reorganisation of the NHS into regional health authorities, the regional structure became the basis for the postgraduate deans' network. Each Deanery established links with the royal college systems of regional specialist advisers and tutors. I first became involved in this system in 1982, as Regional Adviser for my own college, and I remember my first contact with the Postgraduate Dean and GP Adviser through the regular meetings chaired by the former.

Although the Deanery networks expanded locally, the deans and GP advisers were also working at national level and developing a relationship with the Department of Health, which was to become increasingly important and complex for three main reasons. First, money; second, the differing governmental responsibilities for health in England, Scotland, Wales and Northern Ireland; and third, the increasing awareness of medical workforce problems.

During the 1980s, following the Griffiths Report,[1] general management was introduced to the NHS to replace consensus management, typified by the cogwheel system, and NHS funding became more explicit. Budgets were set – if not yet strictly adhered to – and doctors were encouraged to become involved in budget decisions. The separation between the funding of hospital and community services and general medical services extended into PGME and, in particular, in the hospital sector, the financial demands of medical education began to be more difficult to reconcile in a world where service budgets were being set and more closely scrutinised by Government. By 1987, health authorities across the country had serious financial problems: wards were being closed and the level of clinical and public dissatisfaction was growing.

For the deans in England and Wales, the Department of Health and Social Security (DMSS) was the Government department in charge of health administration and funding. This was not the case for Scotland. The national forum at which the deans met the DHSS was the Committee of Postgraduate Medical Deans (COPMED), which had no remit to discuss Scottish matters. There was, in addition, the Conference of Medical Deans and Directors of Postgraduate Medical Education of Universities in the United Kingdom (UK Conference), which was UK-wide, but this was more of an academic and developmental meeting rather than a managerial or policy group. Eventually this situation was resolved, in 1997, by joining the two bodies together to form the Conference of Postgraduate Medical Deans of the United Kingdom (COPMED) and involving all the devolved administrations, not just the Department of Health (DOH). At the same time the regional advisers in general practice became directors of postgraduate general practice, their national forum acronym changing from CRAGPIE to COGPED. The acronyms in medical education are amazing!

In the UK, entry to the medical profession is strictly limited by the availability of medical school places. In England until the 1990s there had only been a small expansion of these places since the origins of the NHS, with only three new medical schools, in Nottingham, Leicester and Southampton, and much of this capacity was based in London. At postgraduate level, control was maintained through the availability of senior registrar posts, a process which, by the 1980s, was the responsibility of the Joint Planning Advisory Committee (JPAC). Through COPMED nationally, and through their own networks locally, the deans were becoming more involved in the management of the tight control of the numbers of hospital doctors. This put the deans at the centre of an increasing conflict between the demands of the NHS for medical staff and the need to provide good quality education. This tension was to increase over the next few years and would bring the deans into conflict with both the NHS locally and with the medical Royal Colleges. The strict control of senior registrar numbers meant that service needs were often met by an expansion in the numbers of senior house officers (SHOs), many of whom were exploited as pairs of hands with poor educational prospects. Too often, overseas-qualified doctors, on whom the NHS depended, filled these posts with little chance of advancement.

Working for Patients

In 1989, *Working for Patients*[2] was published. On the service side it led to the 1990 Health and Community Act, and to the internal market. For education, the key lay in the 10th and final 11th, but unnumbered, working papers. These dealt with non-medical clinical education and with medical and dental postgraduate and continuing medical and dental education, respectively. Where the Christchurch Conference created the postgraduate deanery system, *Working for Patients* proposed that the funds used to support the direct costs of PGME should be identified, taken out of service allocations and the resulting education budgets given to the postgraduate deans to manage through the regional health authorities. These funds covered the basic salaries of trainee doctors, their study leave costs, the running costs of postgraduate centres and libraries locally, and the costs of administering the postgraduate deanery network, including the regional advisers in general practice. Excluded were the costs of CPD for career-grade hospital doctors, and any indirect PGME costs, as well as the GP education costs which were in the general medical services (GMS) budget. In 1992 these proposals were implemented through the executive letter (EL(92)63).

It is difficult to appreciate the impact of this development. When I was appointed Postgraduate Dean for North West Thames in 1991, the department had a budget of approximately £500 000. After EL(92)63 this rose to £47 million. Deans moved from being pastoral co-ordinators of PGME to managing it, with the financial power to force real change. However, they had neither the systems, nor indeed the structures or experience, to manage this responsibility. It changed their relationship with the NHS and moved the centre of gravity of deaneries further towards the NHS and Department of Health. Few realised it at the time, but it made the deans a key instrument of departmental policy.

The influx of earmarked funding did secure real improvements in the infrastructure of PGME, and the control of a significant part of trainees' salaries did enable the deans to improve working conditions and educational opportunities. The financial clout was, however, far better used as a lever to develop sustainable relationships with the new NHS trusts and commissioners, which were being created as part of the internal market. It was important that clinical tutors did not use the new funding to develop a 'state within a state' mentality that could lead to a dangerous isolation of PGME from the general business of the trust. It was all too easy to forget that the ring-fenced PGME funding took no account of a very considerable amount of indirect funding which supported educational activities at local level.

At regional level there was a considerable expansion of deanery posts, with the appointment of business managers to cope with the complexity of managing large budgets and of associate deans and regional advisers, who combined part of their time in the deanery with a continuing career in clinical medicine. The associate deans became involved in specific areas of deanery activity, such as flexible training, overseas doctors, groups of clinical specialities and their associated regional training committees or particular geographical areas within the deanery. Although the administrative costs of these training committees were met by the deanery their success depended on the involvement of consultants, GP principals and trainees. For hospital doctors this involvement required the good will of hospitals, just the type of indirect PGME cost that was not included in deanery budgets. As training became more structured this cost was to become a greater burden on the service and another potential cause of tension between deans and the NHS.

The higher profile that the deans achieved as a result of these changes led to some tension between them and the royal colleges, the joint higher training committees and their specialist advisory committees (SACs), over their respective roles in inspecting training posts and giving them the necessary educational and manpower approval. Lack of effective collaboration in these processes could result in sudden local crises, and in trusts feeling that there was excessive duplication of inspection and insufficient deanery appreciation of the realities of service provision. Since during the general practice element of GP vocational training trainees were supernumary and GP trainers were paid, these issues did not occur. This was not true of the two-year hospital-based component of vocational training.

Individual deaneries developed their own styles and approaches to these issues. Despite their joint accountability to the medical school and to the NHS regional health authorities some deaneries remained firmly based in universities, whereas others moved much more towards the NHS. In 1995, another NHS reorganisation reduced the number of regional health authorities from 14 to eight. The number of deaneries stayed the same, so that in some parts of England two deaneries were linked with one new regional health authority. The following year regional health authorities were abolished and many of their functions, including PGME, were taken into the newly created regional offices of the NHS Executive. The dual accountability of the deans and regional advisers was now to the university and to the Civil Service rather than to the NHS. At the same time the ring-fenced PGME funding held by the deans was consolidated into the new Medical and Dental Education Levy (MADEL), one of the few funding streams that flowed through regional offices as opposed to those of the commissioning health authorities. The deans, as part civil servants holding medical education funding at regional and local levels brought direct Government input closer than ever.

Calman and higher specialist training

At the same time as these changes were taking place, a working group chaired by the Chief Medical Officer for England, Sir Kenneth Calman, reported on the organisation of PGME. His recommendation was for a more structured approach to higher specialist training, with a shorter overall training period leading to a Certificate of Completion of Specialist Training (CCST) granted by a new body, the Specialist Training Authority (STA), which would have a role for specialist training akin to that of the JCPTGP. Whilst the SHO grade would remain unchanged, there would be competitive entry into a new specialist registrar grade that would replace the registrar and senior registrar grades. Each successful entrant would be given a national training number (NTN) and would embark on a structured training programme with a regular review of in-training assessment (RITA). The postgraduate deans would manage recruitment to the grade, the allocation of NTNs and would oversee the RITA process. The royal colleges would produce the training curricula and the joint higher training committees and their SACs would approve training programmes (not just posts). The new system was supposed to be 'cost neutral'. The national decisions on the allocation of NTNs, now the de facto controlling system for consultant numbers, and on their geographical distribution were made by the Specialist Workforce Advisory Group (SWAG) working within the overall strategic framework of the Advisory Group on Medical Education Training and Staffing (AGMETS).

The aim of the Calman Report[3] was to produce a more structured approach to specialist training, with greater consistency in the quality of training and the possibility of shorter training programmes. This was a further step in the move from the apprentice model of medical training. The idea that it could be cost-neutral was unrealistic, and the system came in for some criticism about shortening the length of training time, especially from some surgical specialities, and the effect on academic training. The brunt of implementation, and managing the potential for disruption to service, as programmes were established fell on the deans and emphasised their role as the practical bridge between Government policy on PGME and the NHS. The Calman reforms did not affect the SHO grade directly. Indirectly, however, the concentration on specialist training left many SHO posts in the wilderness of service provision without education, prompting the comment from one dean that SHOs were now a 'lost tribe'.

Consortia, confederations and the isolation of postgraduate medical education: *A Health Service of all the Talents*

Despite an increasing appreciation of the importance of teamworking, and a more multidisciplinary approach to healthcare, PGME has until very recently developed separately and in isolation from the other clinical professions, apart from dentistry. For nursing and the therapies, *Working for Patients* introduced a shift of training from NHS-based schools of nursing and health into higher education, with far less emphasis on postgraduate and post-basic training. In the nursing and therapy professions there is no equivalent to the postgraduate dean to act as a link between education and service. With a few notable exceptions, deans have not paid too much attention to educational links with the other clinical professions.

In 1996, along with the creation of MADEL, a non-medical education and training levy (NMET) was created, through which the central funding for purchasing education for other clinical professions from higher education could be managed. Who would manage it? Local education and training consortia were established, consisting of service providers, who used NHS-trained clinical staff, with the NHS commissioners of service. The guidance for the consortia provided for the involvement of postgraduate deans, but few of them took this up and even fewer deaneries encouraged real joint initiatives. Consortia were only partly successful and, in its 1999 report on NHS staffing requirements, the House of Commons Health Select Committee recommended that there should be a major review of NHS workforce planning.

The acceptance by the Government of this recommendation resulted in the publication, in 2000, of a consultation document *A Health Service of all the Talents: Developing the NHS Workforce.*[4] This document appeared within a few weeks of *The NHS Plan*[5] and its recommendations became a key instrument of the workforce development aspects of *The NHS Plan*. Its terms of reference were to review the workforce planning arrangements for all professional groups within the NHS, and to explore barriers and opportunities for efficient and effective workforce planning in the context of current and known future policy initiatives. It also considered the roles and responsibilities for the workforce at all levels within the NHS and the then NHS Executive.

The recommendations in this consultation document shaped the current pattern of education and workforce development in the NHS. The main considerations were:

- greater integration of training and workforce planning with service policy and delivery
- multidisciplinary workforce planning

- merger of the education and training levies to give integrated funding
- central action to co-ordinate work on skill mixes and new types of healthcare workers
- the establishment of a National Workforce Development Board supported by care group workforce development boards
- chief executives to have responsibility and accountability for workforce plans
- the creation of workforce development confederations to bring together, at local level, NHS and other employers of healthcare staff with education-providers (including the Postgraduate Deans), these would replace the consortia and be more inclusive
- the appointment of regional directors of workforce development to whom postgraduate deans and confederations would report

In addition, a fundamental review of primary care was promised, together with a look at the SHO grade. It was accepted that not only would the number of doctors need to increase, but also that the ways in which they worked would need to change.

Within a year most of these recommendations were being implemented. They were to have, and will continue to have, profound implications for deaneries and the way they work with the NHS. Twenty-seven confederations were in place and, at least notionally, there was a single multiprofessional education and training levy (MPET), of which MADEL was a part. In future, the MPET would be routed through the confederations, and the deans would derive their funding through them and be accountable to them. This was implemented through service-level agreements.

A review of the future operation of NHS education and training funding was set up, which I chaired. Its recommendations formed part of a consultation paper, *Funding Learning and Development for the Healthcare Workforce*, which was published in 2002.[6] A key proposal was that in future budgets should be based on the type of educational activity being supported rather than being based on a specific professional group.

Shifting the balance of power

'Shifting the Balance of Power' was the name given to the programme that aimed to move power in the NHS to local levels and, indeed, to the 'front-line'. The NHS Executive was abolished as a separate entity within the Department of Health. The regional tier of Department of Health management was first reduced from eight regional offices to four 'Directorates of Health and Social Care'. A nice illustration of the inverse relationship between the length and splendour of a title and the transient nature of the position, the directorates lasted just a year before they, too, were abolished and strategic management of the NHS was devolved to 28 strategic health authorities (SHAs), formed in 2001 as part of the same process. Now, some three years later, workforce confederations (now increased to 28 to be coterminous with SHAs) are also being absorbed into them. In the current system the deaneries will be accountable to SHAs and will derive their levy funding from them. For some, such as the Oxford Deanery and Thames Valley SHA, there is a one-to-one relationship. In contrast, in London there is one deanery to five SHAs, and in the West Country two SHAs each have to deal with two deaneries!

The GP directors have also had to face the consequences of change in the NHS with the creation of primary care trusts (PCTs) and teaching PCTs. There is, too, the emphasis on primary care as opposed to general practice. The GP education structure at local level has to interact with the professional structure of local medical committees, and the NHS structure of SHAs, PCTs and, in some cases, teaching PCTs, all of which have their own views and influence on the education process.

The work of deaneries is now concerned as much with workforce issues as with education. In an NHS that is increasingly driven by targets, there has been a focus on the number of clinical professionals, including doctors, and how to increase them in order to improve both access to services and the quality of those services. Consequently, the deans and GP directors have been caught up in a ministerial drive to increase the number of consultants and GPs in the service. The other aspect of work which has increased has concerned the working conditions of trainees, both through the 'New Deal' scheme and the application of the European Directive on Working Hours (EDWH) to trainee doctors. Concerns about bullying and harassment have also become more prominent, and these, as well as the effect of recent race and disability discrimination legislation, will be a source of more complex interactions between the deaneries and the NHS, with the potential for conflict and tension between clinicians and hospital managers.

Paradoxically, the focus on working conditions in general, and the European working time directive in particular, has partly masked appreciation of another major change in the postgraduate medical training system. The 'lost tribe' of SHOs is finally receiving some attention. The consultation document, *Unfinished Business*,[7] the reform of the SHO grade led, in 2003, to *Modernising Medical Careers*.[8] Implementing the changes these documents recommend will be a major task for the deans and a costly one for the NHS, which has not fully woken up to their implications.

The future

We have come a long way in PGME in the past 40 years, much of it in the past 12 years since the publication of EL (92) 63 in 1992. Postgraduate deans started out as a hybrid between the traditional senior clinical academic administrator (as their title suggests) and an educational leader within the NHS. The title remains and some deans and deaneries are still firmly located within the setting of the local university medical school. The reality of funding, and of Governmental expectations, combined with the need for a close working relationship with the NHS means that the balance has shifted decisively towards the NHS. It can be a struggle to maintain the academic side of the job at a time when educational innovation and research and development are so badly needed.

Both deans and deaneries have reacted to a series of NHS- and Government-inspired changes, not all of which have been well thought through. Deans have just been expected to cope. The current structures and approaches do vary from deanery to deanery, for the simple reason that in the UK there has never been a 'root and branch' examination of what it is reasonable for a deanery to do (and, by implication, what is not reasonable), how these functions should be funded and implemented most effectively and efficiently, which personal and organisational skills and competencies are required to do this and how they can be reliably and systematically developed. Time and time again the deans have been given extra duties simply because they are there, without any real thought as to whether they have the skills, the organisation or the funding to do the job. Rarely have they said 'No'. Whenever the question of a thorough review of the deans' function has arisen, the argument has been raised that they are too busy and vital to some new initiative (such as implementing the Calman recommendations) for their work to be disrupted. Viewed in this light, the system has been remarkably resilient and effective. Now, finally, a review is being undertaken and I look forward to seeing what its conclusions will be.

There is a major educational challenge in relation to how doctors in the future will respond to working with the public, with patients and with other clinical professions. We are good at training, the preparation for the known. The challenge lies in medical education: the preparation of doctors for unknown futures in a rapidly changing society where the profession of medicine will need to find a new equilibrium and define a new contract with a more sceptical and less deferential society. My main concern is that the deanery system is properly equipped to play a lead role in working with the NHS to meet this continuing educational challenge.

References

1   Griffiths R (1983) *NHS Management Inquiry: report*. DHSS, London.

2   Department of Health (1989) *Working for Patients*. HMSO, London.

3   Department of Health (1993) *Hospital Doctors' Training for the Future: The report of the Working Group on Specialist Medical Training*. HMSO, London.

4   Department of Health (2000) *A Health Service of All the Talents: Developing the NHS Workforce*. HMSO, London.

CHAPTER 2

Organisations involved in postgraduate medical education and training

Beverley Gainey and Neil Jackson

Introduction

In the modernised National Health Service (NHS) there are now a significant number of organisations other than postgraduate deaneries involved with postgraduate medical and dental education and training. With the deaneries, these allied organisations work together for the common benefit of postgraduate education and training, postgraduate trainees and, most importantly, patients by:

- joint strategic planning
- influencing and lobbying where necessary
- sharing appropriate information and good practice
- delivering key policy areas
- achieving an appropriate balance between service and education
- ensuring quality service for patients through developing a highly trained and committed medical workforce
- ensuring an established learning culture in all NHS organisations
- facilitating the co-ordination of a regional approach to the delivery of postgraduate education and training, such as pan-London
- promoting multiprofessional or multidisciplinary work-based learning.

The main responsibility of postgraduate deaneries is to commission, oversee and monitor the provision of postgraduate education and training for doctors and dentists in NHS training posts. This chapter describes the organisations that deaneries must work with to discharge their many functions.

The organisations involved in postgraduate medical education and training include the following:

- General Medical Council (GMC)
- Postgraduate Medical Education and Training Board (PMETB)
- the royal medical colleges
- the NHS University (NSHU)
- strategic health authorities (SHAs)
- workforce development confederations (became part of the strategic health authorities from April 2004)
- postgraduate deaneries
- NHS trusts
- medical schools
- the National Clinical Assessment Authority (NCAA)

In 2003 there were approximately 37 000 doctors and dentists in England training for careers in general practice, in 70 medical specialities and in nearly 30 sub-specialities. Professor Sir Liam Donaldson, Chief Medical Officer, said in 1999, 'A properly managed and funded system of postgraduate education is vital to ensure that our doctors and dentists are equipped with the knowledge, skills and attitudes they will need to provide a quality service.'[1] The organisations involved in postgraduate education have been subjected to a lot of change in the years following that statement, including boundary changes, the emergence of new organisations, such as workforce development confederations (WDCs) with their subsequent amalgamation into strategic health authorities (SHAs) and the Postgraduate Medical Education and Training Board (PMETB), with changes to funding arrangements and budget structures. The environment in which these organisations operate has changed amid a wealth of initiatives to facilitate a more patient-centred approach to healthcare, to improve the working lives of healthcare workers, to implement the 'European Working Time Directive' and to foster multidisciplinary and interprofessional working and learning. The education path for doctors in training is also changing, with the introduction of foundation programmes followed by a broader specialist programme and subsequent in-depth specialisation, as required. This will replace the current pattern of three training grades.

The General Medical Council

The General Medical Council (GMC) is a body with charitable status, established by an Act of Parliament[2] to 'protect, promote and maintain the health and safety of the public'. The GMC exists to serve the interests of patients and it does this by maintaining registers of persons it deems fit to be medical practitioners, who have demonstrated that they have received an appropriate medical education. Prior to the Medical Act (1983) the GMC discharged its responsibilities through seven statutory committees: Education; Interim Orders; Preliminary Proceedings; Professional Conduct; Assessment Referral; Professional Performance and

Health. These committees were revised in the 1983 Medical Act as follows, i.e. Education, one or more Interim Orders Panels, one or more Registration Decisions Panels, one or more Registration Appeals Panels, the Investigation Committee and one or more Fitness to Practise Panels.

The GMC keeps two registers of medical practitioners. The first is a 'register of medical practitioners' consisting of four lists: the principal list; the overseas list; the visiting overseas doctors list; and the visiting European Economic Area (EEA) practitioners list. All persons on the principal list on the first of January are included in the Medical Register, which is published annually. In addition, the GMC has discretion to publish the Overseas Medical Register in any particular year.

The second register maintained by the GMC is the 'register of medical practitioners with limited registration' for those persons with limited or provisional registration. All medical practitioners must be registered with the GMC on either of these two registers.

The GMC has the power to advise members of the medical profession on standards of professional conduct, professional performance and ethics. Where it considers that the interests of the general public are best served by doing so the GMC will disclose information relating to a practitioner's professional conduct, performance or fitness to practice, for example through ill health. The Professional Conduct Committee has the authority to strike a doctor's name from the register, thereby removing their right to practise medicine. It can also suspend registration pending enquiries or make a person's registration conditional upon compliance with requirements set by the GMC that are either designed to protect the general public or are in the individual's best interest.

The GMC Education Committee exists 'to promote high standards of medical education and to co-ordinate all stages of medical education'. It provides the general public with the assurance that all persons it has included on its register have sufficient education and relevant experience to equip them with the professional knowledge and skills they need to be able to provide a good standard of practice and care to their patients. The Education Committee ensures that each medical practitioner on its register has been educated in the necessary areas of knowledge and skills at an approved institution, to a sufficiently high standard and for an appropriate period of time (at least a six-year course or 5 500 hours of practical and theoretical instruction). It does this by setting out what it requires to be taught in order to obtain primary UK qualifications and by setting the proficiency standard for passing qualifying examinations. It maintains the education and examination standards it has set through examination inspectors and by appointing visitors to medical schools who submit reports to the Education Committee. The Education Committee also determines the patterns of experience that count towards the requirement to fulfil a prescribed period of employment in a resident medical capacity. This includes at least two branches of medicine and it grants where the service, while thus employed, has been satisfactory.

The GMC assesses the education and experience of non-UK graduates to ensure that they are of an equivalent and acceptable standard.

The Postgraduate Medical Education and Training Board

The Postgraduate Medical Education and Training Board (PMETB) was established in 2003 to take up its responsibilities in October 2004 as an independent authority with a statutory remit to supervise postgraduate medical education and training, raising standards and quality wherever possible. The PMETB subsumes the Specialist Training Authority (STA) and the Joint Committee on Postgraduate Training in General Practice (JCPTGP). At the time of publication, however, the PMETB is now set to assume its responsibilities as from September 2005. The PMETB collaborates with the GMC to ensure that there are 'Coherent and continuous arrangements for the entire continuum of medical education'.[3] The GMC continues to have responsibility for undergraduate training while postgraduate dental education remains the responsibility of the General Dental Council (GDC).

The PMETB has 13 medical and 12 lay members and held its first meeting in October 2003. Its primary objectives are the safeguarding of the health and well-being of individuals needing or using the services of a general practitioner (GP) or specialist and ensuring that the standards it sets meet the professional needs of doctors undertaking postgraduate medical education and training.

With the advent of PMETB, the arrangements for general practice and specialist training are combined, bringing together all those parties responsible for postgraduate medical education in the UK and ensuring that their interests are aligned. It works closely with related educational and regulatory bodies, including the medical Royal Colleges and Faculties as these are key elements of the education and training arrangements. The PMETB assesses doctors completing final postgraduate training leading to a Certificate of Completion of Training and allowing inclusion on the Specialist or General Practice Registers.

Medical royal colleges and faculties

There are sixteen medical royal colleges and faculties, reflecting the broad medical specialities, but there are numerous sub-specialities within colleges and faculties. Each royal college is an independent organisation and the Academy of the Medical Royal Colleges co-ordinates the work of these bodies. After successfully completing the training period as a pre-registration house officer (PRHO) a doctor in training obtains full registration with the GMC and can embark on his specialised training, including general practice. Membership of a royal college is then obtained by assessment or examination.

The medical royal colleges and faculties individually determine the essential education that a doctor must acquire in the senior house officer (SHO) grade before they are equipped to begin specialist training. Through a network of regional advisers and college tutors, they give educational approval to posts and training programmes that fulfil the medical college or faculty's curriculum, specifying the knowledge, skills and attitudes that are required and the standard to which they must be attained. Regional advisers liaise with the postgraduate deaneries at a regional level and local college tutors ensure that protected and sufficient postgraduate medical education is in place locally to meet trainees' educational needs.

The educational requirements of specialist registrars (SpRs) are immensely varied as there are a multitude of career paths to the grade and their management arrangements are very complicated. The medical royal colleges and faculties set the standards and assessments to be achieved, although the extent varies by speciality. Management of the separate training programmes is undertaken by the postgraduate deaneries, and the PMETB will issue the Certificate of Completion of Training at the end of training either as an SpR or as a general practice registrar (GPR).

The NHS University

A Health Service of all the Talents[4] documented a mismatch between the needs of the NHS and the investment and priorities of educational providers and professional bodies. The NHS University (NHSU) was set up as an SHA by statute[5] on 1 December 2003 to be a corporate university for all 2.75 million people working in either health or social care in England. As an organisation it represented the embodiment of the premiss that developing individuals professionally and personally translates into developing and improving the service they provide for health or social care patients and clients. It also facilitated life-long learning for all health and social care staff, regardless of how few or many qualifications they already have, and its remit extended to involving patients, carers, volunteers and members of the public. Its initial educational developments include a masters level programme, an NHS induction programme and 'Health Learning Works', which is a scheme whereby long-term unemployed people are assisted into careers in health and social care. The NHSU was aligned to the University of Warwick when established, with nine regional offices, and the intention was to deliver the majority of its programmes locally. To meet an existing unmet need by entering educational provision, it was developing key relationships with partner groups such as WDCs, SHAs, postgraduate deaneries, the royal colleges and professional bodies. It was envisaged that by 2008 it would be fully operational, with university status and offering research and degrees. However, a recent government announcement has confirmed that the

NHSU will be absorbed into a new NHS Institute for Learning, Skills and Innovation (Nilsi) by mid-2005. The new institute will continue to enhance service delivery in the NHS through innovation, learning and leadership and bring together the work already being undertaken by the NHSU, the NHS Modernisation Agency and the NHS Leadership Centre.

Strategic health authorities

SHAs were established in October 2003. There are 28 SHAs and they share the same border alignment with local authorities, which have responsibility for social services. SHAs manage the NHS at the local level on behalf of the Department of Health. The SHAs translate national priorities into local objectives and incorporate them into their local plans for the delivery of healthcare. The SHAs ensure that NHS organisations are working together to achieve the local delivery plan, contributing to the national NHS plan for modernised patient-centred services.

Workforce development confederations/ directorates

SHAs have accomplished their workforce plans and managed the Department of Health's annual investment in training initially through WDCs. These are partnership organisations that were established in April 2001 after consultation on *A Health Service of All the Talents*.[4] From April 2004 WDCs were merged with their local SHAs, by which they had previously been performance-managed through a business plan agreement. WDCs consist of representatives from all local stakeholders, both NHS (trusts, ambulance trusts, primary care trusts, SHAs and postgraduate deaneries) and non-NHS (local authorities, private and voluntary sector providers) to plan and develop the whole healthcare workforce in order to meet the healthcare needs of the local population. The WDCs link closely with further and higher education institutions, the prison service, NHS Direct, learning and skills councils, the Ministry of Defence, the National Blood Service and others. Working together, they carry out a pivotal role in the analysis of the numbers and skill mix of staff required by the stakeholders, now and in the future, as well as the provision of appropriate education and training for all groups of healthcare staff. They also devise and disseminate improved human resource strategies that help to reduce recruitment and retention problems, which enriches the working lives of staff.

WDCs are responsible for the postgraduate medical and dental education of doctors in training. They work in partnership with postgraduate deaneries, through a business plan agreement, to organise the management and provision of postgraduate medical, dental and interprofessional education. The WDCs seek to optimise the use of resources to meet effectively both the needs of the service and the professional needs of postgraduate doctors and dentists.

With the progression of time WDCs have now been incorporated into SHAs as formal workforce development directorates (WDDs).

Postgraduate deaneries

The postgraduate deaneries are members of WDCs, from which they receive their funding. There are 21 postgraduate deaneries in the UK: one each for Wales and Northern Ireland; four for Scotland and 15 for England. A single deanery can relate to more than one WDC and SHA. For example, London is the largest post-graduate deanery and relates to five WDCs or SHAs.

Postgraduate deaneries commission, manage and monitor postgraduate med-icaland dental education to the standards set by the universities, the GMC, the GDC and the PMETB, carrying out this function in the context of *The NHS Plan* and the commitment to multiprofessional working and learning, and to patient-centred care. The deaneries have to make sure that the performance and progress of doctors and dentists in training is reliably and fairly assessed and recorded. They commission NHS trusts and primary care trusts to provide post-graduate medical training. Postgraduate deaneries set up specialist training committees, STCs, and work closely with royal college regional speciality advisers, to make sure that doctors and dentists in training are placed in suit-able working environments, in both secondary and primary care settings, and have regular assessments. Postgraduate deans delegate responsibility for training for general practice to a Dean or to a Director for Postgraduate General Practice Education.

Postgraduate medical deans, directors of postgraduate general practice edu-cation and postgraduate dental deans work collaboratively in respective national groups, that is to say, the Conference of Postgraduate Medical Deans (CoPMeD), the Committee of General Practice Education Directors (COGPED) and the Committee of Postgraduate Dental Dean (COPDenD). All three bodies perform similar national roles. For example, the CoPMeD is where member deans meet to discuss topical issues, to share best practice and to agree a uniform and fair approach to training in all deaneries. It provides a forum where other interested organisations, such as the Department of Health, the BMA or the GMC can meet UK deans.

NHS acute trusts, mental health trusts, community trusts and primary care trusts

Trusts have a contractual responsibility to the postgraduate deaneries to ensure that the doctors and dentists in training it employs receive sufficient quantity and quality of postgraduate education and training. Directors of medical education and clinical tutors are the managers and educationalists at NHS trust level, often based in dedicated education facilities. College tutors, speciality tutors and the body of consultant staff support them in this role. They have a budget determined by their relevant postgraduate deanery and this provides for the education centre, its running costs, the study leave expenses of doctors and dentists in training, and often helps with the running costs of a library.

Primary care trusts (PCTs) are lead NHS organisations in assessing patient need, planning and securing all health services and improving health for their local populations. They are also concerned with the development of all primary care services linked to local workforce development requirements, and they work closely with deaneries with regard to GP recruitment and retention.

Medical schools

In London the medical schools are responsible for the educational well-being of pre-registration house officers (PRHOs)[6] and the trusts are responsible for the delivery of education to those standards. These bodies are monitored by the Postgraduate Dean. Outside London the Postgraduate Dean has total responsibility for the PRHO year.

Royal Colleges

The Royal Colleges are responsible for setting the educational standards pertaining to basic specialist training or general professional training for SHOs and these standards are exercised through college regional advisers and college tutors. The postgraduate deanery is responsible for ensuring that the NHS delivers education to these standards. At trust level the college and clinical tutors, supported by the medical education committee, ensure the appropriate delivery of training. SHO posts are inspected by the Royal Colleges to ensure that they conform to the educational criteria laid down for them.

Postgraduate Medical Education Training – competency standards and supervision

The PMETB (and formerly the Specialist Training Authority and Joint Committee on Postgraduate Training for General Practice (JCPTGP)) is the competent authority to issue a Certificate of Completion of Training to specialist registrars (SpRs) and general practice registrars (GPRs) who have successfully completed their period of training. Before the PMETB was established trainees received a Certificate of Completion of Specialist Training issued by the Specialist Training Authority or a Certificate of prescribed or equivalent experience from the JCPTGP.

The responsibility of the GMC for setting educational standards and determining the curriculum is exercised through the Royal Colleges, through college regional advisers and college tutors, whereas the postgraduate deaneries commission and monitor those standards. The Programme Director is responsible to the STC for the delivery of all the education and training for individual SpRs in their speciality programmes. Trusts and clinical tutors are responsible for the delivery of that portion of the SpRs' training that takes place in their locality, generally lasting 12 months.

The clinical tutor ensures that all grades of doctors and dentists in training have access to induction courses, and that opportunities for career and pastoral counselling are in place. Induction courses are particularly important for PRHOs and all doctors taking up their first UK training placement, but they should be available at the start of any new placement. The clinical tutor also ensures that each doctor and dentist in training has a personal development portfolio and receives appropriate appraisals and assessments.

National Clinical Assessment Authority

The National Clinical Assessment Authority (NCAA) provides support to employers when there are concerns about the performance of an individual doctor or dentist working in an NHS trust, the prison service or the Defence Medical Services. The NCAA will provide advice, take referrals and carry out targeted assessments on doctors and dentists in difficulties, who may be either trainees or established independent doctors. The employing organisation remains responsible for resolving the problem once the NCAA has produced an assessment. Deaneries work closely with the NCAA and employer organisations to provide support and, where necessary, remedial training programmes for doctors who are performing poorly.

Summary

The needs of patients and local communities are paramount in the new NHS, and they must be supported by an appropriate system of planning, educating and developing a multiprofessional or multidisciplinary workforce of healthcare professionals at national and local levels. Postgraduate deaneries and their partner organisations have an important part to play in ensuring that the medical part of the workforce is appropriately recruited, trained and retained to meet the needs of the NHS.

References

1   Chief Medical Officer (2000) *Medical and Dental Education Levy – Accountability Report 1998/ 99.* Crown copyright: Department of Health, London.

2   *Medical Act 1983 (Amendment) Order 2002* (2002) Crown copyright.

3   Liaison Group of the Specialist Training Authority: policy statement (2002) *Taking stock – The Challenges Facing Medical Education and Training Within a Changing NHS*. Specialist Training Authority, London.

4   Secretary of State for Health (2000) *A Health Service of All the Talents: Developing the NHS Workforce*. Crown copyright: Department of Health, London.

5   Statutory Instrument 2003 No. 2772 (2003) *The NHSU (Establishment and Constitution) Order 2003*. Crown copyright.

6   National Association of Clinical Tutors (2000) *Training and Resource Pack*. National Association of Clinical Tutors, London.

CHAPTER 3

Training in the new NHS

Shelley Heard, Wendy Reid and Anne Hastie

Introduction

For many years the way we trained doctors changed very little. Doctors were trained by the apprentice system with attachment to a consultant firm. This was expected to be full-time and often meant working more than 100 hours per week, but this had to change not only for the sake of the trainee but also for the patients. Some of the radical ways that this old system is changing are described in this chapter, dealing with the training programme, the ways of working and the time spent.

Modernising Medical Careers

Modernising Medical Careers[1] was published in February 2003. It was the response from the four UK Secretaries of State for Health to a document published in 2002 by the Chief Medical Officer called *Unfinished Business: Proposals for Reform of the House Officer Grade*, a review of the SHO grade.[2] The review of the early aspects of British postgraduate medical education was promised in *The NHS Plan*[3] laid out by the Government in 2000. The mention of such a review in a high-level policy document such as *The NHS Plan* is indicative of just how important addressing some of the key issues in postgraduate medical education was deemed to be.

Modernising Medical Careers, however, addressed a far wider range of issues than just the SHO grade. It proposed three new strategic directions for British postgraduate medical education:

- the introduction of a foundation programme directly following graduation from medical school
- proposals to consider the development of a 'run-through' grade to encompass both early and late specialist training, with a view to streamlining specialist training to meet the workforce requirements of the NHS
- consideration of how opportunities could be made available to enable doctors

to meet the requirements to enter the specialist register (SpR) grade if they had previously not been able to do so.[4]

Foundation programmes

The introduction of a two-year, competency-assessed programme after graduation from medical schools has three main objectives, which are to:

- ensure that, two years after graduation, doctors have robust and secure clinical skills that enable them to manage safely the acutely ill patient
- integrate these clinical skills with well-developed professional attitudes and behaviours
- offer an opportunity for recently qualified doctors to consider a range of career opportunities to support their own aptitudes and interests while supporting the future workforce requirements of the NHS. This objective needs to take into account the different settings in which healthcare is offered and should support doctors in improving their understanding and contact with both primary and secondary care.

Foundation programmes will commence for all UK medical graduates from August 2005.[5] In addition, non-UK medical graduates who have not yet achieved the standard required for General Medical Council (GMC) limited registration will also undertake foundation programmes. Doctors eligible for limited registration will not need to undertake a two-year programme, but may well wish to consolidate their clinical and professional skills by undertaking the second foundation year.

The first year of the Foundation Programme, F1, will be broadly equivalent to the current pre-registration year and at the current time, registration at the end of that year with the GMC is anticipated, although the GMC is currently consulting about this issue through its document *Modernising the New Doctor*.[6] The purpose of the second foundation year, F2, is: 'to imbue the trainee with basic practical skills and competencies in medicine and will include: clinical skills; effective relationships with patients; high standards in clinical governance and safety; the use of evidence and data; communication, team working, multiprofessional practice; time management and decision making and an effective understanding of the different settings in which medicine is practised.'

The competencies that foundation doctors will need to acquire have now been defined.[7] Assessment strategies are being developed and will need to be agreed by the Postgraduate Medical and Education Training Board (PMETB). Throughout 2004 and 2005 a number of pilots will be run exploring these and other issues. Although these programmes will be implemented from 2005, as in many areas of postgraduate medical education, they will need to be developed and refined as time goes on.

Run-through training

At present doctors undertake a period of basic or general professional training before entering specialist training. They have two competitive hurdles that must be surmounted: the first is to get into basic training, and the second to get into specialist training. The proposals in *Modernising Medical Careers* point to streamlining this process by creating a 'run-through' training grade, which will effectively mean that once taken into a speciality training programme, subject to satisfactory progress, training will be taken all the way through to accreditation.

This requires each speciality to consider its current basic and speciality training provisions. It will enable the royal colleges and faculties, when considering the standards for training and the approach to competency assessment, to re-look at the duration and content of training to ensure that it meets the future needs of the NHS, so that, where appropriate, the duration may be reasonably adjusted and the outcomes reflect better future service provision. One implication of this, for example, may be that more doctors are trained to deliver general, acute care and that specialist (as opposed to speciality training) training is undertaken by a smaller number of people to reflect more realistically the workforce needs of the NHS. However, until the specific details of these changes have been addressed by the royal colleges and ultimately considered by the Postgraduate Medical Education and Training Board (PMETB), which needs to accept or reject the proposals, they remain speculative.

The need for flexibility

Whatever the final details of the training programmes, it is increasingly clear that, in terms of workforce requirements, there is a need for training to be flexible and responsive to technological and organisational requirements. Along with other European workers for example, doctors will be required to comply with the European Working Time Directive. With a change in the demography of the people entering medicine, especially with the entry of an increasing number of women and more doctors overall wishing to work part-time, a more flexible approach to training continues to be required. Indeed, doctors in training programmes need to have the opportunity to consider their career direction and to make changes if appropriate, both for patient care and to meet their own aspirations. The rest of this chapter addresses some of these issues within the changing context of postgraduate medical education.

Flexible training

Flexible training was introduced more than 20 years ago to retain doctors in training who might otherwise have left the profession because of the demands of full-time training. Flexible training may have had a relatively low priority in many deaneries in the past but current recruitment and retention problems have highlighted the need to improve flexible training opportunities.[8]

Eligibility

Doctors of both sexes are eligible for flexible training but they must have well-founded reasons for being unable to work full-time. There are two categories of doctors who are eligible for flexible training:

- Category I: disability or ill-health; responsibility for young children or other dependents
- Category II: personal development, such as sport, religion and parallel careers.

The budget for flexible training is limited and doctors in Category II are unlikely to obtain funding unless funding allocations increase.[9]

Demand for flexible training

The number of applications for flexible training is increasing each year as medical schools expand and the percentage of female doctors increases.[10] Young doctors want a better life–work balance and the new pay deal for flexible trainees made it a financially attractive option.

In 2003 the percentage of flexible trainees across all deaneries was nearly 6% (London had 10%) and accounted for a total of 1 918 trainees, which is an 88% increase in total numbers over six years.[11] The London Deanery has 27% of the total number of flexible trainees and of these 4% are pre-registration house officers (PRHOs), 23% senior house officers (SHOs) and 73% specialist registrars (SpRs). There is considerable variability between specialities, with palliative care and paediatrics having large numbers, whereas surgery has very few.

Funding

Deaneries hold the flexible training budget, based on 0.6 of the basic salary of full-time trainees and this is cash-limited. The basic salary for a hospital flexible trainee is usually passed to the employing trust on a 0.6 basis, although the London Deanery funds the trust on a pro rata basis. However, the new pay deal for flexible trainees[12] gives them a proportionally higher salary and trusts have to fund the additional costs, including out-of-hours payments. This can make the employment of a supernumerary flexible trainee unattractive.

In the case of GP registrars both full- and part-time trainees are paid from the same budget, which makes the situation easier. Part-time GP registrar salaries are calculated on a pro rata basis, unlike their hospital colleagues.

Types of flexible training posts

In the past, most flexible trainees were supernumerary but there is an increasing trend to make them mainstream by working part-time in a full-time post or by slot-sharing. There is little point in a deanery funding a supernumerary flexible training post when there is a vacant, funded, full-time post, and this situation can occur in specialities where posts are difficult to fill, such as psychiatry. Slot-sharing involves placing two flexible trainees into a full-time post and the flexible training budget funding the overlapping sessions, although local more generous funding arrangements may apply to promote this arrangement. This has been particularly successful in paediatrics, where there are a large number of flexible trainees.

All flexible trainees must be appointed in open competition so they are comparable in professional achievements and potential with their full-time colleagues.[13] If trainees apply for a full-time post they do not legally have to declare their intention to work part-time until they have been appointed, although many prefer to mention this in advance.

Educational approval

Educational approval must be obtained for supernumerary flexible training posts on an ad personam basis from the speciality Royal College, usually through the speciality regional adviser. An agreed weekly timetable (clinical and educational) and a named educational supervisor are required. In the case of SHO posts for general practice training the Director of Postgraduate General Practice Education (DPGPE) should provisionally approve the timetable, which must then be sent to the speciality Royal College for educational approval. The DPGPE can then give educational approval on behalf of the Royal College of General Practitioners (RCGP) and this is ratified by the deanery GP Education and Training Committee.

The future of flexible training

As the number of hospital flexible trainees increases, a new approach may be necessary to bring these doctors into mainstream training. There are fewer problems with part-time training in general practice, which is partly due to part-time training being mainstream and funded from the same budget.

European Working Time Directive

The European Working Time Directive is a major challenge for postgraduate medical education.[14] Until the introduction of the Calman reforms to the registrar grade in the mid-1990s it was accepted that training in hospital specialities was by an apprenticeship, with minimal control over the length of time necessary to achieve consultant status. Since the introduction of structured training programmes a number of attempts have been made to reduce the number of hours worked by trainee doctors. The latest legislation of the European Working Time Directive will reduce, stepwise, the average hours of work per week to 48 by 2009. Implementation is a legal requirement for the NHS but it is also a part of the wider aims to improve the work–life balance for NHS staff.

Other workers have been subject to the legislation for some time, but doctors in training were allowed to defer (derogate) adherence to the directive until August 2004 when all doctors in training had to work an average of 58 hours per week with defined rest periods and compensatory rest contracted.

From August 2004 the rest provisions are:

- there must be 11 hours continuous rest in every 24-hour period
- a minimum 20-minute break when shift exceeds six hours
- a minimum 24-hour rest in every seven days
- a minimum 48-hour rest in every 14 days
- a minimum four weeks annual leave.

There have been a number of initiatives resulting in reduced hours of work for junior doctors over the past decade. Running up to the European Working Time Directive was the 'New Deal',[15] which from August 2003, although contracting doctors to 56 hours of work on average per week, has less restrictive requirements for rest periods. The 'New Deal' was managed by many trusts through the mass recruitment of doctors into non-training posts, such as trust doctor or staff grade posts. Increasing the number of doctors working at one grade protected rotas, but training opportunities were diluted and reduced because doctors required the day off after a night on call. The disruption to the long-standing consultant firm was significant, with complex planning of rotas required not only to provide a semblance of continuity of care but also to allow trainees access to their named trainer.

The ruling in the European Working Time Directive that 11 hours in every 24 must be for rest means, realistically, that full shift patterns of work must be introduced. Two rulings by the European Court of Justice are important in the understanding of the European Working Time Directive. The SiMAP ruling followed a Spanish case and states that time spent on-call in a hospital counts as working time, even if the doctor is sleeping. The consequence of this is that being available to work the next day because they have had a quiet night on call is, for many doctors no longer possible as they are deemed to have been working. At the moment there is a review of the second European Court of Justice ruling, the Jaeger case, which requires compensatory rest to be taken in the next shift or period of time worked. Obviously, this would have devastating consequences for the service if doctors are required to take, for example, four hours out of a shift because the previous day an emergency had required them to work through their breaks and into the 11 hours of rest required. Once clarification of the Jaeger case is received the full impact of the compensatory rest requirements can be calculated.

In January 2003 the Department of Health issued guidance (HSC 2003/001) about the European Working Time Directive, which detailed the requirements for August 2004 and included information from a number of pilot sites across the UK. It made suggestions for developing an action plan (*see* www.doh.gov.uk/workingtime/).

The broad headings are:

- reduction in the number of rotas by employing cross cover and reducing the number of tiers available
- new working patterns, implementing broader teams to cover the hospital at night and developing new roles for non-medical staff
- expansion of staff numbers with a planned expansion in the consultant workforce to enable a move towards a consultant-delivered service; SpR grade numbers to be released to allow for this rather than an expansion in the number of trust doctors
- teamworking, with effective use of non-medical practitioners, such as night nurse practitioners
- new service models, starting from the premiss of the need to maintain local access to services wherever possible and also to improve the quality of patient care
- use of information technology.

As well as the pilot sites, a number of other hospitals have reported on their initial experience in introducing European Working Time Directive-compliant patterns of care. Great Ormond Street[16] and the Royal Free hospitals in London have contributed to the pool of experience by developing night teams to provide out-of-hours cover across the specialities. The Great Ormond Street (a specialist paediatric hospital) model, although not widely applicable to acute trusts providing both adult and paediatric services, provides a number of useful lessons for those trusts moving towards new working practices. Of particular interest is the enhanced role for senior nurses, leading the clinical night team, and the importance of careful audit of activity before new patterns of work are introduced.

The hospital at night

The concept of the 'hospital at night' was first suggested by Professor Elisabeth Paice in 2001. Working differently at night relieves the pressure on daytime staff, releases more trainees for daytime hours and therefore improves access to training opportunities. The development of a team of healthcare professionals to provide out-of-hours care for patients is complex. It is not sufficient to pool a number of doctors together and call them a team. The structure and content of the team needs to reflect the case mix and the complexity of the clinical workload, the grades of the trainees available and their individual training needs. It would be unreasonable, for example, for an obstetric SpR to cover trauma and orthopaedics. Similarly, although the planning for a night team is difficult and fraught with tensions between specialities, it is vital that those who develop different strategies for patient care are flexible and able to think 'outside the box'. The imperatives of patient safety and delivering quality care will drive the need for audit and standard setting for new models of care.

Many hospitals are now developing the 'hospital at night' concept: each will be different, as each trust will have a different set of service requirements and different resources.[17] The inevitability of full-shift working for doctors in training requires accepting the fact that shifts are unpopular if they occur too frequently at night. Pooling the number of doctors at night to provide a generic team competent to manage the out-of-hours workload, well supported by non-medical healthcare professionals allows for improved patient care, permits better continuity of care by allowing for scheduled documented hand-overs, the development of teamworking skills and leadership skills as well as reducing the number of nights an individual doctor would have to work if covering a single 'firm' or consultant workload as in the past. Of course, this is a radical change away from the single consultant firm, with its widening-towards-the-base pyramid of juniors and a hierarchical view of delivering patient care. However, with the challenges facing medical education today, not least the European Working Time Directive, new ways of working need to be embraced if we are to improve the standards of patient care and maintain the quality of postgraduate training.

Conclusion

So we have seen that the way and the environment in which we train our doctors are changing for the benefit of the trainees and our patients. This should not, however, be seen as the end of the story as training will continue to change as a response to changes within, and needs of, the healthcare system of the country.

References

1   Department of Health (2003) *Modernising Medical Careers. The Response of the Four UK Health Ministers to the Consultation on Unfinished Business: Proposals for Reform of the House Officer Grade.* Department of Health, London. (www.mmc.nhs.uk/keyarticles/FINAL_VERSION_UK_POLICY_STA.PDF)

2   Sir Liam Donaldson, CMO (2002) *Unfinished Business: Proposals for Reform of the House Officer Grade.* Department of Health, London. (www.mmc.nhs.uk/keyarticles/SHOREPORT.PDF)

3   Department of Health (2000) *NHS Plan: A Plan for Investment, A Plan for Reform.* DoH, London. (www.publications.doh.gov.uk/nhsplan/nhsplan.htm)

4   Department of Health (2003) *Choice and Opportunity: Modernising Medical Careers for Non-consultant Career Grade Doctors.* Department of Health, London. (www.mmc.nhs.uk/keyarticles/MODERNISING_MED_CAREERS_NCC.PDF)

5   Department of Health (2004) *MMC: The Next Steps – The Future Shape of Foundation, Specialist and General Practice Training Programmes.* Department of Health, London. (www.mmc.nhs.uk/keyarticles/NEXT_STEPS_FUTURE_FOUND-SPEC-GP.PDF)

6   General Medical Council (2004) *Modernising the New Doctor: Consultation on the Review of PRHO Training.* General Medical Council, London. (www.gmc-uk.org/med_ed/default.htm)

7   Academy of Royal Colleges Working Party (2004) *Core Competencies for the Second Foundation Year* (draft). Academy of Royal Colleges, London.

8   Department of Health (2001) *Improving Working Lives Standard.* Department of Health, London.

9   Conference of Postgraduate Medical Deans (2000) *Eligibility for Flexible Training.* COPMED, London.

10 Allen I (1994) *Doctors and Their Training: A New Generation.* Policy Studies Institute, London.

11 COPMED Flexible Training Working Group (2003) *Analysis of 2002/2003 Annual Survey.* COPMED, London.

12 Department of Health (2000) *Modernising Pay and Contracts for Hospital Doctors and Dentists in Training.* Department of Health, London.

13 Goldberg I and Paice E (1999) Flexible specialist training compared with full-time training. *Hospital Medicine.* **60**: 286–9.

14 Department of Health (2003) *The European Working Time Directive, Guidance.* Department of Health, London. (www.doh.gov.uk/workingtime/)

15 NHS Management Executive (1991) *Junior Doctors – The New Deal.* Department of Health, London.

16 Cass H D, Smith I, Unthank C *et al.* (2003) Improving compliance with requirements on junior doctors' hours. *BMJ* **327**: 270–3.

17 NHS Modernising Agency Hospital at Night (2003) (www.modern.nhs.uk/hospitalatnight)

CHAPTER 4

Teaching the teachers in primary care

Robert Clarke

Introduction

This chapter explores the value of educational theory for the preparation of teachers in primary care. Teaching encompasses a range of methods for facilitating learning. To help the development of new teachers, this complexity needs to be addressed within a supportive yet challenging learning environment. One example of a teaching programme is discussed in detail, in which course days are held once per month over a 10-month period. The peer support provided by this format is a key component in developing reflective educational practice.

Modelling

Preparing primary care practitioners for a teaching role is an exciting challenge, particularly as the participants will almost certainly model the methods used in the teaching programme as they develop their own teaching practice. This means that course tutors need to imagine that they have two heads. One head is engaged with running the course and the other is involved in reflection to ensure that learning activities are congruent with the stated course ethos – to encourage adult learning. In other words, there is a symmetry within 'teaching the teachers' which is aptly summed up by 'do as you would be done by' or, better, 'teach as you would be taught'.

Adult learning is most effective when it is clearly relevant to the reality of working life, relates theory to practical problem-solving and encourages reflection.[1] All of these components need to be considered by the teaching team.

What sort of teacher?

When vocational training for general practice was introduced in the UK, the

Royal College of General Practitioners (RCGP) published a book, *The Future General Practitioner*.[2] This extended the role of a teacher by going beyond the traditional method of passing on knowledge. Additional teaching methods were explored, in which the teacher was seen as a facilitator of learning through questioning, promoting autonomy in the learner and encouraging self-discovery and reflective practice. The four main teaching methods are summarised in Table 4.1, where the role of the teacher and links with other writers are indicated. The Socratic approach involves helping leaners to become aware of the limits of their knowledge or their implicit values and beliefs through asking awareness-raising questions.[3] Heuristic teaching methods aim to encourage discovery learning. This respects the autonomy of the learner, a key component of learning theory, in which learning from experience is promoted.[4,5] Reflective practice fits well with counselling styles of teaching in which the teacher's role is to promote the exploration of feelings, self-discovery and the examination of implicit assumptions.[6-11]

Table 4.1: Teaching methods and the teacher's role

Teaching method	Main process	Role of teacher	Links with authors
Didactic	Telling	Passing on knowledge	Discussed by many authors
Socratic	Questioning	Facilitating learning through awareness-raising questions	Neighbour[3]
Heuristic	Encouraging discovery learning	Promoting learner autonomy and self-directed learning	Kolb[5], Knowles[4] Brookfield[1]
Counselling	Exploring feelings and assumptions	Encouraging self-awareness, self-discovery and reflective practice through exploring feelings and examining assumptions	Schon[9], Heron[6] Lave[10], Bolton[7]

This broader view of education means that the process of preparing practitioners for a teaching role is complex. The strong parallels between the practitioner–patient relationship and the teacher–learner relationship soon become obvious to those taking up this challenge. This helps with both understanding and motivation. Many practitioners report that their preparation to become a teacher is an excellent form of continuing professional development because it influences behaviour in the consulting room and extends the range of interventions used with patients.[12] It also helps learners to explore their own learning styles, making real and personal the link between teaching, the promotion of learning and the implicit assumptions of each learner.[8]

Course formats

Preparing practitioners for a teaching role involves a number of possible components:

- introduction to educational theory, including curriculum planning, teaching methods, learning styles and assessment
- teaching practice with learners, including teaching communication skills and clinical topics
- educational theory and its application in real life; development and assessment of teaching skills
- peer support in development as a teacher, including problem-based learning.

A variety of preparatory programmes exist. On one hand, some offer short introductions (for example, two to four days) with an overview of educational theory and then introduce practitioners to practical work with learners, with ongoing supervision and support. This sometimes takes place in a facilitated learning set. Alternatively, theoretical components can be presented and discussed over separate course days in a modular format.

The 'Teaching The Teachers' (TTT) course, based in London, provides a 10-month university-accredited course, that leads to a postgraduate certificate for teachers in primary care. A two-day introduction is followed by monthly course days. This course is intentionally non-modular so that people are unable to opt in and out of the course, the result being that a constant peer group works together over the entire course. This arrangement has been found to be very powerful, mirroring the process that exists between learners and individual teachers in primary care. Aspects of this course are described in detail in this chapter as one example of an effective programme.

Generic teachers' course

As primary care has developed, practitioners are increasingly engaged in collaborative working with other professionals, and some practices have set themselves the explicit task of striving to become learning organisations.[13] For this reason, TTT became an interprofessional course seven years ago, and focuses on the core skills of teaching required by practitioners from medical, nursing and complementary medicine backgrounds. This means that some additional role-specific training may be required as well as the main programme. A uniprofessional example is given in Figure 4.1. A doctor wishing to become an undergraduate teacher may wish to attend a module on clinical skills teaching, whereas a postgraduate trainer will need a 'nuts and bolts' course to cover the regulations governing GP registrars, and a potential course organiser may attend a course specifically designed to teach group skills.

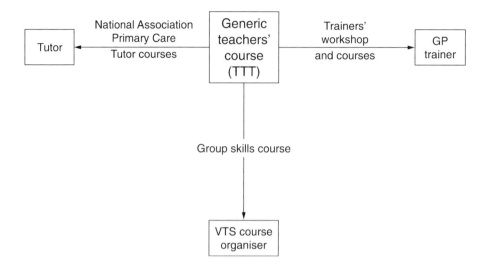

Figure 4.1 Examples of role-specific pathways.

Selection

Attending the TTT course is a prerequisite to becoming a GP trainer, but it is not the final selection process. In other words, this is a necessary but not sufficient preparation for becoming a trainer. The ethos of general practice and the facilities, including library, information technology (IT) and clinical records, must also be assessed on a training practice approval visit.

For potential GP trainers, TTT is a stage of selection on the path to becoming a trainer. About five years ago, two criteria for joining the course were introduced. First, all GP applicants must have completed the Membership of the Royal College of General Practitioners (MRCGP) examination. Where exceptions to this criterion have been made, individuals have struggled with the work involved, because MRCGP is required to become a trainer and it has been difficult for learners to do both their teaching work and their MRCGP preparation properly. Second, potential learners have to attend one of three open evenings held each year. Here, the TTT leaders give an outline of the programme, clarifying the amount of time involved and providing an opportunity for potential students to ask questions. It is also the start of the process of small group work, which is tried out with specific tasks. Doing this enables the course leaders to assess whether this method of working will suit each individual. On some occasions, group leaders have been able to predict that an individual may find collaborative working a challenge but have nevertheless decided to accept that student. On others, individuals have been 'unable to attend an open evening'. Of the few occasions when there have been significant problems with learners, almost all have been from a group that did not attend an open evening.

Personal tutor

Each learner is allocated a personal tutor, who normally leads the small group of which he or she is a member. The personal tutor is available for informal support and discussion throughout the TTT course. In addition to pastoral care, the tutor reads and gives feedback on two formative essays, aiming to ensure that each learner is familiar with critical, reflective and academic writing, including referencing conventions, by the time the end-of-course assignments are written. Students are given individual written feedback with an invitation to discuss this in detail at the next course day. Providing feedback is very time-consuming for tutors, but is felt to be a key opportunity for formative feedback and is greatly appreciated by students. At least two formal tutorials are offered, lasting about 20 minutes each, and normally following the written feedback on the formative essays. If a student fails one of the final assignments, the personal tutor offers a meeting and will provide support in resubmitting the referred work. Students are encouraged to seek advice informally at coffee breaks and lunchtimes, and tutors' e-mail addresses (as well as work and home telephone numbers) are freely available from the start of the course.

Curriculum

The TTT course is a generic course for teachers in primary care within the National Health Service (NHS). It is suitable for all primary healthcare practitioners who see patients as part of their work. The common needs of these practitioners are emphasised, and include:

- the need to analyse and teach communication between practitioner and patient, including clinical issues
- the need to learn and teach evidence-based healthcare
- the need to work and communicate effectively in interprofessional primary care teams.

The aims of the TTT curriculum are to meet the broad educational needs of all teachers in primary care by critically evaluating:

- the principles of education
- work-based self-directed learning
- self- and peer-assessment for continuing professional development.

The aims are linked to the following intended learning outcomes. Learners should be able to:

- design a curriculum appropriate to the needs of learners
- analyse a range of educational methods and relate them to the principles of learning
- critically evaluate the ability to provide learning support
- identify and critically evaluate a range of assessment techniques and select and use them appropriately
- reflect on learning and develop a critical inquiry approach to teaching practice
- communicate effectively with learners and with peers
- plan and critically evaluate personal educational goals in the context of the needs of the organisation.

The core philosophy underpinning the TTT course emphasises a partnership model, encouraging collaboration between and among tutors and students, with active encouragement of self-directed learning. Interprofessional learning, portfolio-based learning and tutorials (in both small group and one-to-one with the personal tutor situations) encourage the integration of theory with practice.

The delivery of the TTT curriculum is unusual by comparison with most university courses. It involves a close partnership with students. Not only is the ordering of topics on course days varied, but the content of each day varies according to the needs and wishes of the students. University accreditation of this learning model was a particular challenge because of this flexibility, but was established on the basis of the examples from previous years. Similarly, the list of topics given in Table 4.2 are examples from a typical year. The course leaders aim to promote 'learner-centredness' in those they train, and the process of having a dialogue about the course curriculum is an essential component of the TTT programme.

There is a tension between a completely learner-centred approach and an approach that is based on a structured syllabus. This is the same tension that is

Table 4.2: Example of a TTT course outline

1	Introduction: teamwork
2	Introduction: teaching communication skills
3	Curriculum planning
4	Teaching practice 1
5	Practice visits – peer review
6	Assessment
7	Teaching practice 2
8	Student-determined topic (for example, teaching time management)
9	Student-determined topic (for example, teaching critical appraisal)
10	Student-determined topic (for example, clinical supervision and mentorship)
11	Open space technology
12	'Teaching assignment'

experienced by teachers in primary care, who are keen to facilitate the self-directed professional development of those they are teaching and yet are aware of the very real and specific needs of the service. The TTT course leaders attempt to strike a balance, supporting the group within the course aims and intended learning outcomes.

In practice, each course day is planned two months in advance. Normally, about three-quarters of the topics are constant from one year to the next. Student representatives are appointed early on, and a formal meeting takes place every few months. They have provided valuable feedback. Minutes of meetings are circulated to all, and contribute to the participatory ethos of the TTT course.

The introduction to the course comprises two consecutive days, in which teamwork exercises are started. On the second day, communication skills teaching is introduced, with actors starting the process of exploration of different models of the consultation and, more importantly, different models of teaching.[14, 15] A month later, the third course day focuses on curriculum planning.

There are 12 course days, held approximately once per month. Between course days, learners are expected to spend a minimum of one day in private study and a minimum of one day in work-based activity, for example peer review on visits to other students' practices and reflection on how course themes apply in students' own practices. Many students spend considerably more time than the minimum and they sometimes complain that the course involves too much hard work. However, by the end of the TTT course, most learners appreciate the benefits of the self-directed approach, and the same holds true when student views have been surveyed some time after the course has been completed.

On each course day there is large group discussion, and various tasks related to the topic of the day take place in the morning. In the afternoon, learners break into their tutor groups, where communication skills work, hot topics and reflection on the themes of the day are encouraged.

Subsequent course days occur at monthly intervals and usually include learning styles, teaching methods, teaching practice with volunteer learners, formative assessment and giving feedback, as well as topics suggested by the learners.

The important point to note is that there is flexibility to respond to student need. Some students feel anxious or 'lost' at the beginning of the TTT course when they realise that there is no rigid timetable of topics, but they soon appreciate the benefits of a flexible timetable: their views are taken into account; there is discussion of the course direction on each course day; and they share responsibility in partnership with the course tutors

The final course day is the teaching assignment, in which each learner has to lead a teaching session for his tutor group. The tutors rotate for marking purposes and there is an external examiner in each group. Students are encouraged to mark each other to gain familiarity with a specific construct-based marking tool. These marks are not actually used but it is an opportunity to use the assignment for further learning about the process of assessment. The TTT curriculum is intended to help students develop key skills.

Communication skills

Students are expected to communicate effectively about teaching and learning in written and group work.

Intellectual skills

Students are able to analyse and critically evaluate different theoretical perspectives, and explore the relationship between theory and practice.

Teaching skills

By the end of the course, students should be able to facilitate learning in both one-to-one and group settings.

Independent work and group work

Students should be able to manage time effectively, should interact effectively with their group and need minimal help in directing their own learning. They will be able to support each other, recognising and evaluating the different roles within a team, including reflecting on their own preferred roles and collaborating across interprofessional boundaries.

Self-evaluation

Students are expected to evaluate their own strengths and weaknesses, as teachers and as team members, applying their own judgements both confidently and sensitively. They will be able to make effective use of reflective practice, including reflection on their effectiveness as educators.

Interprofessional learning

Multiprofessional learning occurs when groups of different professionals attend the same course. *Interprofessional* learning means more: here, there is an explicit aim to examine each others' roles in order to improve collaborative practice.[16-18] This interprofessional focus has been very successful, with GPs valuing the model of reflective practice developed by nurses, and primary care nurses reporting how much they have benefited from using the consultation-skills approach developed by GPs. Learning together enhances effectiveness in working together, and improves patient care and fits in with the recent emphasis on teamwork in the NHS.

The composition of the teaching team is diverse and interprofessional, in keeping with the TTT course philosophy. Because the course is interprofessional, the course tutors pay particular attention to mixing students from different professional groups. Interprofessional 'pride and prejudice' arises inevitably between the different professional tribes, and can be used as a basis for experiential learning. Once such issues have surfaced, groups usually decide to devote a session to an explicit exploration of this area, which the flexible timetable easily accommodates. This aspect of the TTT course has been greatly valued by students.

In order to encourage interprofessional participation, the course has recruited using a 'buy-one-get-one-free' approach. In previous years, the TTT team noted several occasions on which GPs had attended and enjoyed the course so much that they encouraged their practice nurses to attend in subsequent years. It would have been even better if the two had attended together – as an interprofessional pair. Encouraging interprofessional pairs from the same practice to attend together was used as a marketing strategy. Nevertheless, there have been real challenges in recruiting nurses. Some nurse managers have regarded the course with suspicion and perceived it as doctor-led and doctor-dominated because it is organised and funded by a GP department.

Throughout the programme there is an emphasis on peer-group support and interprofessional teamwork, which is as important in learning as it is in service delivery. Small-group work is used to create a co-operative learning environment in which safety is used as a foundation for challenge, constructive feedback and critical reflection. This process is fostered by the integral, one-year format of the course.

Practice visits: peer review

On one of the course days, each of the small groups of eight students and one tutor meets separately at one of the students' practices. This is intended to serve as a model of how peer review can be facilitated.[19] Following the taught day, students visit each other's practices (usually based on locality) in groups of three and conduct their own peer review process. They are encouraged to write up their observations for the benefit of each other and to keep such written reflections in their portfolios.

Formative assessment

On each course day, there is protected time spent on reflective practice in small groups, facilitated by the course leaders. In addition, students are set two essays on key topics. These essays are voluntary. Course leaders provide written feedback to those who choose to submit them. The subjects will vary depending on the needs of the group, for example previous topics have included:

- an essay on curriculum planning
- an essay on teaching methods and learning styles.

These assessments are considered to be important in facilitating learning but do not count towards the final grade awarded. The topics chosen are directly relevant to the end-of-course assignments, and previous students have found feedback from tutors helpful in preparing them to write their final assignments.

Summative assessments

There are two written assignments and one small-group teaching session:

- a case study
- a critical analysis of the participant's personal development plan (PDP)
- teaching assignment.

The assignments are designed to be as useful as possible for a new teacher, who will have to design a curriculum and help learners with their own personal development plans. In addition, it is important to assess teaching directly, otherwise the course risks becoming overly academic. Examples of recent assignments include the following.

Case study (3000-word essay)
You will be asked to design a learning environment with appropriate identification of educational methods and learning support mechanisms, justified with critical reference to course material and the literature.
A health professional who has been out of practice for seven years has decided to return to his or her previous clinical role in primary care. His or her professional qualifications remain accepted by the accrediting bodies. You have agreed to take him or her for six months of re-orientation and training. Discuss your approach with critical reference to educational theory.

Personal development plan (PDP) (1500-word essay)
Write a critique of your personal development plan. Please provide an outline of your existing PDP as an appendix, which *will not* be marked and *will not* be included in the word count.

Teaching assignment (small-group teaching session)
You will be asked to:
  - facilitate learning in the group about a topic of your choice demonstrating core course themes. You will have a total time of 20 minutes.

The TTT course leader team meets to mark the final assignments. The teaching assignment is led by each student in his or her tutor group. The tutors rotate to different groups, and each group also has an external marker with previous knowledge of the TTT course. The session is videotaped so that the team of examiners may review any borderline cases. These include those on the pass/

merit and merit/distinction boundaries as well as those who are borderline pass/ fail. A selection is made available to the university liaison tutor and to the external examiner.

The two written assignments are 'marked residentially', in that the course leader team meets for two days. This allows a calibration exercise for each assignment and for double marking, with discussion and moderation where significant differences are noted.

Staff development

The whole TTT course leader team recognised that there were interprofessional issues for teachers as well as for students. The team therefore attended an experiential one-week module 'Organisational Life: Pride and Prejudice in Interprofessional Work'. This stimulated the development of new approaches, which have been used on the TTT course. For example, the course leaders are now much more aware of interprofessional tension when it arises and therefore are more likely to draw attention to it. This stimulates new insights and sensitivities in students, which usually leads to a request to devote a course day to further exploration of this important aspect of professional life.[20, 21]

After the course

A year after the TTT course, the vast majority of students are engaged in and developing new educational roles within primary care. Two previous students have become TTT course leaders in subsequent years. Many course participants have applied to become GP trainers. This involves a peer review visit to their practice and an assessment of their skills as a teacher against national criteria. A review of reports from one area showed the high levels achieved by students. Not all students are successful at their first attempt – this depends partly on the amount of additional work they have done outside the course days.

Conclusions

Preparing practitioners for a teaching role in primary care is a challenging but rewarding task. Current models of education view teachers as facilitators of learning rather than the traditional passer-on of knowledge and skills. This preparation requires a preparatory 'teaching the teachers' course which should use the same teaching methods and ethos that we expect from students once they develop their own teaching role. The key qualities of such a course are its flexibility, its learner-centredness and its ability to encourage students' self-discovery, autonomy and continuing development as teachers. Ideally, a course of this type should take place over a relatively long period of time, to allow the establishment of a supportive and trusting peer group. With this basis, students can engage in reflective educational practice, not only improving their teaching skills but also questioning and challenging their own assumptions.

Acknowledgements

This chapter has been translated and published as an article in a Polish medical journal. The author would like to thank the TTT course leader team for its support and collaboration in developing the programme and stimulating the development of ideas expressed in this chapter. The team includes Arnold Desser, Christine Menzies, Mandy Platts, Nicky Poulain and Andrew Wilson.

References

1 Brookfield S (1986) *Understanding and Facilitating Adult Learning: a comprehensive analysis of principles and effective practices*. Open University Press, Milton Keynes.

2 Royal College of General Practitioners (1972) *The Future General Practitioner: learning and teaching*. British Medical Journal, London.

3 Neighbour R (1992) *The Inner Apprentice*. Petroc, Newbury.

4 Knowles M (1990) *The Adult Learner: a neglected species*. (4e). Gulf Publishing, Houston.

5 Kolb D (1984) *Experiential Learning*. Prentice Hall, New Jersey.

6 Heron J (1989) *The Facilitator's Handbook*. Kogan Page, London.

7 Bolton G (2001) *Reflective Practice: writing and professional Development*. Paul Chapman Publishing, London.

8 Claxton G (1996) Implicit theories of learning. In: Claxton G, Atkinson T, Osborn M, Wallace M (eds) *Liberating the Learner*. Routledge, London.

9 Schon D (1987) *Educating the Reflective Practitioner*. Jossey-Bass, San Fransisco.

10 Lave J and Wenger E (1991) *Situated Learning: legitimate peripheral participation*. Cambridge University Press, Cambridge.

11 Bion W (1961) *Experiences in Groups*. Routledge, London.

12 Heron J (1990) *Helping the Client: a creative practical guide*. Sage Publications, London.

13 Senge P (1990) *The Fifth Discipline: the art and practise of the learning organization*. Doubleday, New York.

14 Pendleton D, Schofield T, Tate P *et al.* (1984) *The Consultation: an approach to learning and teaching*. Oxford University Press, Oxford.

15 Silverman J, Kurtz S, Draper J (1996) The Calgary–Cambridge approach to communication skills teaching: agenda-led outcome based analysis. *Education for General Practice*. 7: 288–99.

16 Barr H, Hammick M, Koppel I *et al.* (1999) Evaluating interprofessional education. *British Educational Research Journal*. 25: 533–44.

17 Zwanenstein M, Atkins J, Barr H *et al.* (1999) A systematic review of interprofessional education. *Journal of Interprofessional Care*. 13: 417–24.

18 Salmon D and Jones M (2001) Shaping the interprofessional agenda: a study examining qualified nurses' perceptions of learning with others. *Nurse Education Today.* **21**: 18–25.

19 Hasler J (1997) Peer review through practice visits. In: Pendleton D, Hasler J (eds) *Professional Development in General Practice*. Oxford University Press, Oxford.

20 Menzies Lyth I (1989) A personal review of group experiences. In: Menzies Lyth I (ed.) *The Dynamics of the Social. Selected Essays* Volume 2. Free Association Press, London.

21 Halton W (1994) Some unconscious aspects of organisational life: contributions from psychoanalysis. In: Obolzer A and Zagier Roberts V (eds) *The Unconscious at Work*. Routledge, London.

CHAPTER 5

Teaching the teachers in secondary care

Ian Curran and John Krapez

'Personally, I'm always ready to learn, although I do not always like being taught'
(Winston Churchill)

Introduction

To older generations of consultants, being trained and taught were things that happened to you as a junior doctor. Once you had been appointed to your senior post, you learnt from your own experience, from reading the literature, attending conferences and occasionally from remarks made by your colleagues. Little was organised, and serendipity was the order of the day. Moreover, it was, and to some extent still is, assumed by the NHS that as a high value professional practitioner you would automatically be equipped with the wide range of non-technical skills required by the organisation. These high value, advanced professional meta-competencies included the ability to teach, lead teams, communicate effectively, manage and develop services, and guide professional development of both individuals and teams. This wishful thinking on the part of the organisation was seldom justified. In the 1990s with the advent of more objective, structured and transparent training programmes introduced under the Calman reforms it became evident that there were considerable deficiencies in postgraduate training. The challenges exposed by and since Calman can be broadly divided into three areas: knowledge, technical and non-technical skill domains. These challenges place unique demands on both trainees and trainers. An important and difficult area of training provision is within the more nebulous, humanities-based, non-technical skills-based arena.

The non-technical skills, or professional meta-competencies, include areas of practice such as effective communication, teamworking, crisis management, decision-making and conflict management, mentorship and appraisal training, effective teaching, educational supervision and the management of poor performers. This substantial list is far from exhaustive. Furthermore, these skills are becoming increasingly important as the healthcare environment grows more demanding and challenging. This situation has been compounded by frequent and ever more demanding postgraduate reforms, with the result that the previously amateur approach to postgraduate medical education has been rendered obsolete.

Detailed dissection of the constant challenges faced by medical professionals in their daily duties goes some way to appreciate the fundamental complexity of their role. It also highlights the wide range of skills required for competent professional practice. The inherent weaknesses of the existing systems of professional postgraduate development for senior doctors led to the introduction of continuing medical education (CME) by the royal colleges. The demands of clinical governance and a more quality-based, patient-centred agenda have put further demands on an already overstretched senior workforce. Engaging these highly intelligent, busy, professional people in the concept of personal professional development is both challenging and rewarding. Those charged with delivering clinical postgraduate training must develop relevant, focused, engaging learning material if these individuals are to attend. The clinicians generally cannot be compelled to attend and consequently it must be the relevance and quality of the learning material that attracts them to further training. A mandatory requirement for those delivering postgraduate medical education must be to develop a better insight into the adult educational process if they are to develop effective teaching programmes.

Historically, the delivery of knowledge and technical skills training, such as resuscitation training, has been well established for many years. The more complex non-technical skills objectives, however, are a more recent addition to the training portfolio. These demanding training objectives have also proved difficult to deliver because of the fundamental complexity of these higher areas of practice. They have required a fresh and novel approach to training exploring issues such as communication, teamworking and crisis management. At their core, such techniques include challenging behaviour and modulating clinicians' beliefs and performance. Uncomfortable territory for those not trained to do so! Although challenging to deliver, it is essential these high value professional meta-competencies are addressed in terms of training delivery if a quality, patient-centred healthcare service is to develop.

Delivery of high-quality teaching and training is currently metered against by several factors. The constantly changing socio-political backdrop means clinicians expend increasingly significant amounts of effort simply keeping the clinical service going. It is against this onerous and shifting clinical landscape that postgraduate education and training has to be seen in context. Postgraduate education is also currently experiencing an unparalleled level of reform and change. Individual elements of the reforms taken in isolation have very many strengths and potential benefits; however, the scale of the reforms and the haste in their implementation without due consideration to resources and development of trainers may prove overambitious and damaging in the long term.

Recent and future developments, such as the New Deal, the European Working Time Directive and Modernising Medical Careers,[1] have legitimate discrete objectives but their effect on trainee experience has already been considerable. The impact on training in the longer term remains uncertain.

The dramatically shortened specialist training precipitated by Calman and the European Working Time Directive has led to a significant reduction in total training time, from approximately 30 000 hours to perhaps as low eventually as 8 000 hours. This will mean that the quality of training must be enhanced if acceptable levels of performance are to be delivered across the workforce. There is also inconsistency in the quality and content of postgraduate training across the UK; this is counterproductive to career development. The introduction of more objective, better-structured, competency-based training as proposed in *Unfinished Business*[2] represents a potentially significant step forward, but the delivery of this challenging training portfolio will require a level of postgraduate teaching and training hitherto unseen in this country. Central to the success of this initiative will be the development of trainers who are capable of not only delivering the training but also assessing and quality assuring that training. This enhanced training will need to be more effectively delivered than previously. This will require trainers with hitherto unseen levels of insight into the adult educational process. The lack of a theoretical educational knowledge base behind the enthusiastic approach of many hospital teachers contrasts starkly with general practice. The educational work and responsibilities of general practice trainers are underpinned by many excellent educational development courses, often provided on a regional basis. Correcting this fundamental deficiency in hospital practice will require a major initiative among NHS trusts, deaneries and the strategic health authorities. Addressing the core educational deficiencies of the trainers is the first step in creating the right organisational environment to support professional learning and hence develop and enhance best clinical practice.

A raft of Government initiatives, such as 'The Learning Organisation' will founder if individuals are not equipped with the core non-technical skills. Developing reflective practitioners with better insight into non-technical issues such as risk management, decision-making and effective teamworking is essential for these Government initiatives to succeed. Generally, aspects of knowledge and technical skills-based training are usually more straightforward and intuitive; an intravenous cannulation course or endoscopic surgery course is self-explanatory. They are also perhaps more readily understood in terms of training programme delivery, the learning objectives being overt and obvious. A more vexing challenge to training delivery is how, as an educational leader, one addresses learning needs attendant with complex professional behaviour. The tendency to deliver simple courses and programmes that address knowledge and technical skills-based training, often at the expense of the more complex, high-value professional meta-competencies, is perhaps because non-technical skills training is more difficult and far less precise in outcome. A communication skills course may not reform a poor communicator overnight, but when one is exploring poor behaviour a prerequisite to change is often the need to challenge the beliefs and values of the individual. It can be difficult to change the bad habits of a lifetime as they may be deeply engrained. There is, however, obvious value in trying to help a poor communicator be more aware of how to communicate more effectively. Surely it has to be better to try than not to bother at all. To quote Derek Bok: 'If you think education is expensive try ignorance'. A common cause of patient complaints within the NHS is poor communication; it would clearly be unwise to ignore these difficult non-technical areas.

The development of an individual's non-technical skills portfolio is therefore essential if that worker is to practise as a professional rather than a technician. Professionals require insight into the complexity of decision-making attendant with the natural complexity of their role. Put simply, professionals manage chaos. Technicians follow protocols and things are usually black and white; consequently, they tend to be far less flexible. In many areas of healthcare the organisation needs professionals to manage the many grey areas.

This chapter draws on the authors' experience of delivering a wide range of educational courses to hospital practitioners, outlining where possible the key principles and practical points. They also highlight some of the challenges encountered, and discuss issues and areas for potential future development.

Challenges and opportunities

The majority of hospital doctors are enthusiastic and hard-working. They enjoy their work and herein lays the first and most significant challenge to developing educational programmes: how do you get them to realise that there is much that they do not know but which they need to know in order to become better trainers and practitioners? General practice approaches this problem by clearly demarcating between general practice trainers and 'service' general practitioners (GPs). The training process for general practice trainers is highly structured, with a mandatory training course of often 10 days or more. General practice trainer obligations and specific responsibilities are transparent, and there are specific career enhancements and financial rewards to recognise the added commitment, effort and expertise they require. Contrast this with the situation in hospital practice. Trainers in hospital practice are rarely afforded the opportunity to develop as a teacher. There is scant regard, recognition and reward for hospital trainers. Indeed, training could be considered the 'Cinderella' to the two 'Ugly Sisters' of service and research. The new consultant contract, however, brings with it an opportunity to formally recognise the important but often neglected contribution that training makes to healthcare service provision. Teaching and training are as much core NHS business as is service, for without training there will be no service development and quality-enhancement of future patient care. Therefore recognising the importance of training in an organisation is imperative. Without training receiving its due profile and resources, optimal clinical services cannot be developed.

Getting 'training the trainers' right is fundamental to the success of the training reforms such as foundation programmes and competency-based training, which are being introduced by the Department of Health. It is vital that protected time is incorporated and clearly demarcated within the new consultant contract for this increased training burden. If this training time is not duly allocated, the time-sensitive nature of the contract will further erode the status of teachers and marginalize training in general. This further loss of training status is particularly hazardous at a time when the danger of inadequate training caused by shortened training times has never been greater. There is therefore an urgent need for the professionalisation of hospital postgraduate training. This means training trainers to specified levels of competence and recognising their extra skills and responsibilities. This will require the identification and development of 'educational leads' with the necessary educational insight as well as the recognition of other supported trainers who will require allocated time for their training activities. The educational needs of the organisation are now too important to be treated in the previous amateur way. Professionalisation of training activity must be established in hospital practice, as this is the precursor to creating the right learning environment necessary for the development of robust, objective training environments. Organisations will find it difficult to flourish if they fail to invest in the development of their workforce.

A further challenge is presented by the diverse commitments that most consultants manage to sustain. They find it difficult to allocate time to courses lasting more than two or three days and either do not attend them or else ask that they are condensed and compacted. Such requests may, in part, reflect a lack of understanding of the complexities involved or may simply be due to a wish merely to go through the motions in a 'tick-box' fashion. Clearly, the motivation for attending a course is the sole preserve of the delegate, but in this context a clearly communicated prospectus of learning objectives in conjunction with a flexible methodology of course delivery is more likely to engage learners and produce meaningful learning. However, this degree of organisation may of itself fatally undermine the impact of learning if attendees are allowed little time to reflect on their experience and are afforded insufficient opportunity to practise new and perhaps difficult techniques such as facilitation skills. Similarly, reflective practice, a cornerstone of good clinical governance and risk management, is a learnt skill and can only be nurtured if adequate time is made available for it. Creating time to reflect on one's practice or learn is a major challenge for many busy hospital consultants.

The learning organisation

This concept, with its emphasis on the ability of an institution to develop and make progress based on its own experiences, is a powerful driver at the local level to 'Teaching the Teacher' programmes. Technological advances, public expectations and a patient-centred philosophy are also important factors in their development. Career moves by established consultants, once a rarity and viewed with more than a little suspicion, are increasingly the norm, and would-be ship changers are beginning to realise that a well-balanced portfolio of continuing educational professional development, including teaching and training education, is a powerful bargaining chip in the appointment interview.

Modern hospitals are highly complex working environments that demand a flair for a professional role from their senior medical staff. It is vital that they see themselves as professionals rather than technicians, and it is equally important that the hospital management understands the distinction, inconvenient though it may sometimes be. This approach brings with it the requirement to attend meaningfully to professional development. These new challenges require an educational strategy that illuminates the processes of teaching and training complex professional skills. Consultants are increasingly finding themselves the recipients rather than the providers of education. Once the seniors are engaged in ongoing educational demands and are involved in the reflective development of an organisation you are one step closer to a truly meaningful learning organisation. It is then but a small step for senior staff to identify their own learning needs and become truly lifelong learners. This development of a self-sustaining, responsive, reflective organisation is the reward for the investment in training. There is also at its root a key principle that, through effective education, performance can be enhanced. The specious notion that people intrinsically possess all the skills they will ever require is simply not valid. Organisational investment in training and education therefore become the only meaningful alternatives. To illustrate this, consider the old notion that good teachers are born rather than made, and that teaching is essentially something that is intuitive. Although it remains true that a 'natural' will always teach well, even the least-gifted of us can be brought to a satisfactory level by well thought out training and the high flier will perform even better than they otherwise would. The fundamental objective should be the development of a reflective, insightful practitioner who can identify and manage his or her own lifelong learning needs.

Content of teaching programmes

Professional clinical practice can be broadly separated into the following areas. Professionals require an underpinning knowledge base, a technical skills base and an overarching portfolio of professional behaviour and clinical judgement. The training provision of each of these elements present very different challenges and may be considered under the separate headings of specific knowledge, technical skills and non-technical skills.

Specific knowledge

Fortunately, the didactic, fact or knowledge-based course has almost been assigned to the educational dustbin of antiquity. Dry, 'matter-of-fact' pedagogic teaching material is often the learning equivalent of dust and provides little educational sustenance. Knowledge or facts in isolation are largely meaningless. Clearly, a knowledge base is essential to any area of practice but knowledge is far more valuable once it has been put into context. More insightful educational courses use a blended approach, where knowledge is introduced in context and consolidated in a more meaningful learning framework of skills and judgements. With the constant evolution of knowledge and the ever-increasing speed of its propagation, knowledge is no longer the given absolute it once was. It is therefore essential to develop insight into the limitations of knowledge as well as the technical skills required to access up-to-date information efficiently in the Internet age. Managing uncertainty and adopting, where possible, an evidence-based approach are also important emerging themes. Increasingly, it appears more important to know what we *don't* know rather than what we *do* know. This aspect of dealing with uncertainty has a particularly profound importance when exploring how people make decisions with incomplete information – a not infrequent clinical situation.

Technical skills

The Royal College of Surgeons has been especially prominent in the development of programmes for teaching technical skills, borne on the twin pressures of fast-evolving technology and closer scrutiny by an increasingly watchful public. Particular focus has been given to endoscopic surgery since this has the potential to reduce patient morbidity and length of hospital stay, but the technique carries serious risks if performed by those not fully versed in its use. Video has been a particularly valuable tool, whether pre-recorded or via two-way live link, or for the individual working alongside an expert using a camera and visual display unit.

Medicine has adopted training techniques used in other high-risk industries. Virtual reality surgical simulators are now very sophisticated and are capable of taking novices to a high level of expertise before allowing them to apply their skills to patients. The public generally is uncomfortable with the notion that trainees 'practise' on them as patients. While there will always be a 'first time' for every clinician, there is profound logic in having explored many of the basic skills and challenges on a simulated patient before the first live one. Direct supervision for technical skills training remains imperative initially, becoming more distant as competence is achieved. This pragmatic risk-managed approach must represent the best way forward. Simulators have a much wider role to play than merely teaching hand–eye co-ordination and manual dexterity, and they are therefore discussed in greater depth elsewhere in this chapter.

Outside the surgical specialities, the breadth of technical skills training available to consultants is substantial and increasing. From advanced life support refresher training to training in transoesophageal echocardiography, there is now a wide variety of skills training available to senior staff and uptake is reassuringly high.

Non-technical skills

The prominence of non-technical skills in the consultant's range of abilities has been a particular feature of hospital practice in the last 15 years. The increasing involvement of senior medical staff in management, the requirements placed on consultants by reforms of postgraduate medical education (especially Calman) and the younger age and therefore lower experience of consultants on appointment have together spawned a dramatic increase in the need to teach such non-technical skills to senior staff.

For the more senior consultants, who were drawn into management posts following the Griffiths report,[3] formal education in leadership skills, managing change, conflict resolution, employment law, time management and communication skills required a major shift in emphasis from the part-time, amateur approach to something more robust. Most, if not all, of the original training material was derived from non-healthcare organisations. However, much adaptation, improvisation and improvement has taken place since then and it would now be unthinkable for any consultant to take on a clinical director or medical director post without a substantial underpinning from the many organisations offering training and education in the skills and knowledge required to discharge the role successfully. A similar situation exists for clinical tutors, with excellent courses run regularly by the National Association of Clinical Tutors (NACT). Although not strictly 'teachers' in the accepted sense of postgraduate education, such individuals are usually in positions of educational leadership and have a pivotal role in educational development for trainees and trainers. At a trust level their potential impact upon education and training must be a matter of interest and concern for all. Ensuring that clinical managers have a proper perspective on the importance of teaching and training is arguably more important than teaching the teachers themselves, as a hostile clinical service environment can severely jeopardise quality training.

Changing educational needs were not only confined to the upper echelons of NHS trusts and their educational management. Consultants who had hitherto enjoyed a somewhat distant and paternalistic relationship with their trainees suddenly found themselves being asked to appraise them and perform much more structured objective assessments than the traditional 'seems like a good chap' end-of-post report. It was also clear that the reduced length of specialist training introduced by the Calman reforms meant that training needed to be more focused and structured; for many teachers, this would necessitate instruction in how to organise and better deliver training. Pioneer workers, such as Bulstrode, created useful algorithms and methodologies for approaching training in a much less hit-and-miss fashion.

The first surveys of consultants' non-technical skills placed appraisal training firmly atop the list, and a number of training courses – national, local and Internet-based – were established in response. The success of those courses is evidenced in the most recent surveys, in which appraisal training is now bottom of the consultant's learning needs 'wish-list', whereas managing poor performers is at number one. There is an irresistible logic in this which runs thus: we never bothered to look too closely at our trainees; someone told us we had to appraise them; we were taught how to appraise; through our new skill we discovered that some of our trainees have serious deficiencies; help! How do we deal with this? As powerful an argument for teaching teachers as one could wish for and further confirmation of the value of training to the organisation.

Teaching of other non-technical skills has also developed apace. Interviewing and being interviewed, how to teach, performing good research, facilitating, communicating and mentoring are good examples of generic skills that are invaluable to the modern, team-oriented clinician. The situation is anything but static, with new developments continually requiring review and adaptation. A good example of this is the role of appraisal. Originally introduced into hospital medicine as a personal developmental, education-based tool for trainees, the process when applied to consultants quickly became more performance-related, with revalidation turning it effectively into a form of performance assessment. Mentoring is now filling the personal developmental gap thus created, the essential tenets of which are largely indistinguishable from those of the original developmental appraisal. Accordingly, training courses in mentoring for consultants are increasingly being developed.

The role of simulation in training

Airlines and most passengers would consider certifiable anyone who suggested that a pilot, however experienced, should be allowed to fly a passenger-carrying aeroplane without having undergone a period of training on a simulator. The use of aircraft simulators allows a pilot to be tested in safety drills and skills. They are also formally assessed on a regular basis. If they fail they are 'grounded' until such time as they pass. Complex and awe-inspiring though a jumbo jet may be, it is as a toy compared to the intricacies of the human body. Furthermore, aircraft are all man-made; they predictably obey rules of physics and operate in ways which are totally, or very nearly so, under our control. Human bodies answer to a far higher authority and our knowledge of their inner workings remains superficial in many areas. It is little wonder then that simulators have been much slower to establish themselves within the medical profession. However, recent years have seen the development of high-fidelity medical simulators that are capable of accurately reproducing the responses of the human body to physiological insult and subsequent pharmacological intervention. Such simulators constitute powerful teaching tools for trainees and teachers alike. There is also a range of medium- and low-fidelity simulators that also have versatile training roles.

Surgical simulators have been pioneered in the UK by workers such as Darzi and provide valuable technical skills training in technique, particularly for endoscopic surgery. While classified as low to medium fidelity, they nonetheless give an extremely realistic representation of the surgical field. They can be used to provide basic instruction to trainees and, at a higher level, to teachers and trainers. They have particular value in teaching newly developed techniques to senior staff, where adequate experience can be acquired quickly and in relative ease without risk to patients, enabling the 'pupil' in turn to become the 'teacher' to his or her own trainees. This idea of 'co-existent learner and trainer' in the same individual embodies the ideal of practitioners who are both sensitive to their own learning needs and yet capable of training their own trainees and being able to manage their own lifelong learning within an organisational training framework.

High-fidelity simulators come into their own in the field of non-technical skills training. Although they are capable of delivering 'drills and skills' instruction in technical areas, crucially, they can also be used through simulated scenarios to explore more complex skills, such as teamworking, decision making, crisis management and effective communication. It is these high value areas that are of particular interest in training trainers, since these individuals are frequently clinical team leaders. The aviation and nuclear industries realised some time ago that human factors and failure of teamworking were often significant factors in the propagation of disasters. Simulation-based training in these industries has led to an increased awareness of risk management and enhanced industry safety. Similar benefits can potentially be afforded to healthcare through the use of simulators and behavioural debriefs. The value of the use of video feedback in the context of a simulated patient scenario to explore decision-making, actions and how personal performance could have been optimised makes the simulator a powerful tool in developing insight into one's own non-technical performance. The facilitated behavioural debrief by trained facilitators allows participants to explore their thoughts and responses to complex simulated patient-safe situations.

One of the key elements of high-fidelity simulation is that it allows people, through realistic scenarios, video technology and skilled facilitation, to reflect on their own behaviour – together very powerful change agents. A good way to explore a person's behaviour is to explore what they were thinking and feeling; by challenging and possibly changing these thoughts and feelings it is possible to induce long-term changes in behaviour. Consider 'drink-driving' campaigns as an example of this type of behaviour-modifying educational philosophy.

Another significant benefit of facilitation training among facilitators is the heightened level of awareness of risk management in their own clinical practice. In addition, when exploring how trainees develop their own professional identity, role modelling of seniors plays an important part. Having seniors with insight into their own non-technical skills and who are able to 'practise what they preach' creates a strong and desirable training environment. Simulators can therefore help senior clinicians to refine further their non-technical clinical practice and work more effectively in a team. Simulators can potentially play an enormous and important role in clinical risk management training.

Simulators can also serve a valuable role in updating teachers' clinical abilities, by allowing them to be put through a variety of scenarios and ensuring that they are still 'up to speed'. They are of particular value when dealing with rare or dangerous conditions that carry a high real patient mortality if not treated quickly, for example anaphylactic shock. Simulators may also have a role in the assessment and management of poor performers, but the systems have not as yet been adequately validated to allow their use in a situation that could potentially strip someone of their right to practice.

Delivering teaching to teachers

The motivation of busy clinicians to attend training courses can pose serious difficulties that must not be underestimated. Consultants will inevitably 'rank' what they perceive to be the worth of any educational course or meeting against the value that they place on their other activities. If they do not judge the balance to be correct, they will not attend. Other important and powerful motivators include organisational champions, figureheads who can facilitate, support and recognise the value of training within the organisation. Emphasising the relationship between better training and better patient care is essential. Those charged with developing training material must challenge the organisational culture and become educational or training advocates. Showing how the acquisition of a particular skill or insight can be of clinical value to fellow consultants and trainees can enhance this. Needless to say, sticks may sometimes be needed in addition to carrots and the threat of loss of trainees or of training status are extremely effective, if punitive, drivers. Whatever approach is used, it will be time- and resource-consuming, but this is effort well spent. Putting large amounts of energy and resources into creating a course or training programme will be of little value if few trainers enrol.

Dealing with time constraints may require splitting courses into self-contained, half-day bites that can be repeated frequently, not being overambitious with content and polling a selected target audience to determine the optimum timing. It is particularly valuable to enrol the help of the trust management, since it may cancel service commitments for would-be delegates if a sufficiently persuasive argument can be made, especially where clinical teams are concerned. Whatever approaches are used, adequate notice is essential to allow for rescheduling of commitments; advertising and enrolling six months or more ahead of time should be routine. Also, the development of rolling three-, four- or five-year programmes with themed threads, such as teaching, management or professional aspects of practice, is helpful to give structure to the training.

Another important issue is that there needs to be an appropriate number of facilitators and presenters to put on a course. Many local teaching events can be adequately managed with just one or two individuals (two is better, alternating delivery to maintain interest), but others have much heavier requirements if optimum results are to be achieved, especially in the realms of non-technical skills training where small group work is required. A typical example would be with video-consultations for communication training. Any course in which role-playing is a component ideally needs one facilitator for each subgroup. Leaving delegates on their own in a separate room to stumble through a given, or even worse, self-created scenario is simply asking for poor results and disillusioned participants. Facilitators, of course, do not grow on trees; they have to be well-trained and are subject to the same or tighter time constraints as delegates. However, the value of role play is so great in teaching non-technical skills such as appraisal or mentoring that it is well worth the effort and trouble, even if courses need to be limited in number to maintain the correct facilitator: delegate ratio. The value of good-quality facilitators and trainers within an organisation cannot be underestimated. Good training can enhance an organisation's public and professional reputation, which has many potential advantages, including recruitment, staff retention, staff morale and delivering cutting edge innovation in clinical practice.

Conclusion

Some of the challenges inherent in organising and delivering courses for teachers have been referred to above. The authors' experience has clearly taught that engaging and motivating senior clinicians to attend is the most important factor. Delivering high quality, relevant and engaging programmes is essential for high uptake. The benefits to the organisation of developing the non-technical skills base within its senior corpus is essential if a quality, patient-centred healthcare system is to emerge. Recognising the value and necessity of training has never been more acute as in this climate of shortened, time-limited training. NHS trusts, the royal colleges and those charged with delivering postgraduate education must not underestimate the size of the challenge faced, but the opportunities for the future are tantalising. Recognising that trainers need time to train and to learn is imperative if the rapidly changing demands placed upon them by the healthcare system are to be satisfactorily delivered.

References

1 Department of Health (2003) *Modernising Medical Careers.* Department of Health, London. (www.doh.gov.uk/publications)

2 Department of Health (2002) *Unfinished Business.* Department of Health, London. (www.doh.gov.uk/publications)

3 House of Commons Social Services Committee (1984) *Griffiths NHS Management Inquiry Report.* HMSO, London.

Further reading

- Brookfield SD (1991) *Understanding and Facilitating Adult Learning: a comprehensive analysis of principles and effective practices.* Jossey-Bass, Milton Keynes.

- Jarvis P (1994) *Adult and Continuing Education* (2e). Routledge, London.

- Jarvis P, Holford J and Griffin C (2003) *The Theory and Practice of Learning.* Kogan Page, London.

- Handy C (1987) *Understanding Organisations* (3e). Penguin, London.

- Schon DA (1983) *The Reflective Practitioner.* Arena, London.

CHAPTER 6

Induction

Yong-Lock Ong and Suzanne Savage

Introduction

Induction is the foundation on which any job is built and the potential to perform effectively is greatly enhanced if the induction is good. Since the Standing Committee on Postgraduate Medical and Dental Education (SCOPE) report,[1] published in 1993, the NHS has recognised the importance of this process, and induction programmes are now the norm for training posts.[2] In 1997 the General Medical Council (GMC) made it mandatory for all preregistration house officers (PRHOs) to receive induction, and other medical appointments now have induction structures in place, run by trusts and individual departments. The 'Modernising Medical Careers' (MMC) initiative also stipulates that appropriate induction procedures will have to be met.

In 2000 the Department of Health encouraged deaneries to create central induction programmes for overseas doctors, in order to inform these doctors about the UK system.[3] Overseas doctors form approximately one-third of the medical workforce at junior grade, and their distress, misery, homesickness and resentment[4] was thought to spring from unresolved ambiguities embedded in the fine grain of culture and language, in addition to a lack of understanding of what training and working in the NHS is like for everybody.[5]

There is currently great variation in the style and structure of induction programmes, which might include a mixture of lectures, demonstrations and interactive group sessions. Studies on the induction received by new doctors tends to support the use of a staged approach to induction, backed up by comprehensive written information. New doctors do not want all the information about a post at once.[6]

This chapter describes the different induction processes for the various grades and specific groups of doctors, within both hospital and primary care.

Induction for hospital doctors

Pre-registration house officers

The importance of induction for PRHOs is now well established. Induction allows PRHOs to meet members of various hospital disciplines and services, and helps to orient these new doctors to their place of work. An innovative programme has been developed in the eastern region of Scotland for PRHOs taking up posts in the Dundee Teaching Hospitals NHS Trust, by incorporating paper-based patient management problems in the induction programme. With the support of healthcare team members and laboratory staff, patient management problems (describing likely case histories with tasks mirroring the junior doctor's forthcoming responsibilities) have been evaluated as a valuable learning experience. The doctors have quickly learnt how to interact with appropriate hospital staff when managing patients.[7]

Senior house officers

A survey of senior house officers' (SHOs) early induction needs were found to focus on their request for information that enabled them to undertake their service work efficiently and effectively. Information related to clinical education and training could be provided after they had been in post for a couple of weeks.[8]

Overseas doctors

Programmes designed to meet the needs of local graduates do not, however, meet the additional needs of overseas doctors at basic training grade. Based on evidence gained from programmes carried out in Australia, Canada and the USA[9,10,11] the Overseas Deans' subgroup of the Conference of Postgraduate Medical Deans (COPMED) has designed induction programmes for overseas doctors to meet the needs of being new to the country, its medical system and its culture and philosophy. An evaluation carried out on 124 overseas doctors from 43 countries, who undertook the London Deanery induction programme, showed that most participants found the course helpful.[12] A detailed breakdown on the course items (tables 6.1–6.5) gives a clear impression of the items the doctors felt were helpful. Their comments have helped the London Deanery team to refine the content of current courses, focusing on new topics identified and replacing less popular items.

Table 6.1: The NHS

Topic	Usefulness of session (score out of 5)
Clinical governance and the values of NHS	4.2
Informed consent and legal issues	4.6
Postgraduate education and permit-free training	4.6
General Medical Council registration regulations	4.3

Table 6.2: Communication skills

Topic	Usefulness of session (score out of 5)
Defining issues and sharing insights	4.0
Breaking bad news, role play with actors	4.3
Informal medical English	4.2

Table 6.3: Preparing for the next post

Topic	Usefulness of session (score out of 5)
Medicine and the Internet	4.0
Good practice: video and discussion	3.9
Curriculum vitae writing	4.5
Getting on – guest lecturer	4.1

Table 6.4: Multicultural issues

Topic	Usefulness of session (score out of 5)
Working in a multicultural environment	4.1
Doctors working abroad – an English specialist registrar in Africa and an Asian specialist registrar in London	3.9
Death and dying in different cultures	4.3
British reserve – myth or reality?	4.2

Table 6.5: Overall evaluation of the course

Question	Score out of 5
How far did the course meet your expectations?	4.6
How far did the course meet your needs?	4.4
How relevant was the course content?	4.6
How appropriate was the pact of the course for you?	4.3
How much did you enjoy the course?	4.8

European Union (EU) trainee doctors

A smaller study of EU trainees highlighted that their induction needs were different from overseas doctors. They requested topics on informal medical English, obtaining informed consent and other legal issues, role play with actors in a scenario of breaking bad news and an explanation of postgraduate education and training in the UK.[13]

Refugee doctors

The majority of refugee doctors have difficulty being appointed to their first job because they have usually been out of medicine for some time. This absence often varies between three and 10 years, and refugee doctors require help with interview skills and writing curriculum vitae. As part of their extended induction to gain substantive posts in the UK, structured clinical attachments[14] and supernumerary postings have proved helpful in improving their clinical skills and enabling them to establish their medical careers here.

Specialist registrars and consultants

The specialist registrar (SpR) is a higher training grade and the induction of these doctors requires a local introduction to the trusts they work for, to enable them to settle quickly and efficiently into their new postings. Of particular importance is the need for exposure to management issues, and shadowing senior managers can help to create awareness of the management aspects required in various services as preparation for consultant duties. It is also helpful for SpRs to be reminded at induction of an aim to produce publications from their research and special interest sessions. Management and research topics are currently dealt with by a central induction day or half-day programme, provided by programme directors of rotational schemes, to supplement local induction.

Consultants

New consultants report positive benefit from attending an induction programme. This feedback has been consistent among new consultants who have attended the London Deanery 'New Consultant Day' programmes, which are held twice a year. Topics for the day include learning about leadership skills and strategies, developing appropriate negotiation techniques in handling colleagues and sharing early experiences as a consultant.

The recruitment of overseas doctors to consultant grade demands a more extensive induction programme. The programme should include core topics of the structure and values of the NHS, including clinical governance, the GMC regulations on good medical practice, continuing professional development, consultant appraisal and the role of the multidisciplinary team. Local induction at trust level should include the senior doctor's on-call responsibilities, and human resources departments should give help on personal issues such as starting a bank account, driving with a valid licence, registering themselves and their families with a GP (as primary care often has a different role in their countries of origin) and housing and schooling advice.

Induction for general practice

Induction for general practice also follows the principles that have been outlined for hospital doctors, with specific processes applying to specific groups. The induction of a GP registrar starting the one-year period in a training practice, having completed two years of recognised hospital posts, will necessarily be different from that of an EU or refugee doctor being introduced to NHS general practice. Returners to general practice, retainees and flexible career scheme doctors are other groups who require a carefully planned induction, as will any locum joining a practice.

Registrars

In the present system, a registrar joins a training practice that has met prescribed standards laid down by the Joint Committee of Postgraduate Training for General Practice (JCPTGP) and a trainer who has also been approved, using the prescribed criteria.[15] The trainer will normally have attended an approved trainers' course and obtained a certificate of education from a recognised university. 'Trainer' is an unfortunate term as it implies that the registrar emerges 'trained'. In reality, training is a continuous tension between helping registrars to jump through the hoops of summative assessment while preparing them for what will be a lifelong journey of education and practice. The induction programme needs to include a clear structure for the organisation of the year, including a description of – and time for – the assessment processes. It will also need to establish the trainer in the role of facilitator, mentor and educational supervision, as appropriate. The unique and envied one-to-one relationship can then be fully utilised.

Structure of the induction programme

The induction programme would include a written timetable of where and what registrars are expected to do in their first two to four weeks in the practice (Table 6.6).

Table 6.6: Specimen timetable for registrar induction

	Monday	Tuesday	Wednesday	Thursday	Friday
			Week 1		
Registrar (am)	1 Meet trainer for coffee, tour and introductions; 2 Meet practice manager re contract, P45 etc.	1 Computer training; 2 Health visitor clinic	1 Sit in surgery with trainer	1 First tutorial; 2 Computer training	1 Sit in with practice nurse – clinic and treatment room
Trainer (am)	As above	Surgery	Surgery with registrar	1 First tutorial; 2 Short surgery	Surgery
Lunch		PHCT meeting			Partners' meeting
Registrar (pm)	Reception to see how patients access services	Half-day release	1 Computer training; 2 Surgery with trainer	Educational half-day – read protocols, etc.	Half-day
Trainer (pm)	Surgery	Surgery	Surgery	Surgery	Half-day
			Week 2		
	Monday	Tuesday	Wednesday	Thursday	Friday
Registrar (am)	District nurse visits	Video – first consultations (if wished)	Sit in surgery with partner A	1 Short surgery; 2 Tutorial	Sit in surgery with partner B
Trainer (am)	Surgery	Surgery	Surgery	1 Short surgery; 2 Tutorial	Surgery
Lunch		PHCT/business			
Registrar (pm)	Own surgery (half-hour bookings)	Half-day release	Sit in surgery with trainer (joint surgery)	1 Educational half-day; 2 CPN visiting	Half-day
Trainer (pm)	Surgery	Surgery	Surgery	Surgery	Half-day

PHCT = primary healthcare trust.
NB. Some registrars may wish to see patients on their own earlier in the induction.

Ideally, both trainer and registrar meet before the post starts in order to agree the timetable and start to establish a relationship. The induction timetable needs to be shared with all members of the practice team and drawing this up is a good way to ensure their active involvement in the training. The registrar's past clinical experience needs to be taken into account and shared with the team, which may draw on this as a clinical resource. It is important for registrars to be formally introduced to all the members of the primary care team as soon as they join the practice.

The induction timetable will normally include periods when registrars 'sit-in' with different people within the primary care team. It is important that objectives or learning outcomes are understood by both the registrar and the person with whom they are sitting, so trainers have an educational responsibility to set up these attachments appropriately. For both parties, guidance about sitting in has the potential to increase the value of the experience:

- Negotiate what you both want to get out of the session.
- Decide how the person sitting in is going to be introduced.
- Be clear about how interactive the sitter in will be, that is, will he or she examine patients, take histories, etc.
- Check that both parties are both confident and competent to do whatever is decided.
- Give enough time to discuss issues, either as they arise, or collect them to be discussed at the end of the session.
- Ask the sitter-in how he or she is going to record information and questions. If they want to take notes it is usually best to do this after the patient has left the room, or at least to ask the patient for permission to do this.
- Leave enough time at the end of the session for feedback as to whether the learning needs of the sitter-in were achieved.
- If appropriate, feedback to the sitter-in about his or her input.

The induction timetable should include an introduction to the protocols that the practice works to. Use of the computer will also need to be introduced early, as this is the recording method in practices not only for clinical episodes but also for coded data required by the primary care trust to demonstrate compliance with the new general medical service and personal medical service contracts.

In the first few weeks the registrar will need to sign an employment contract. Model contracts can be downloaded from most postgraduate GP deanery websites (*see* www.londondeanery.ac.uk).

According to their degree of confidence, registrars will want the opportunity to see their own patients early on, but unlike the induction of SHOs, the process usually takes place over a period of several weeks rather than days. As the registrar is supernumerary, his or her workload is gradually increased over the year with the aim of managing a 'normal' workload by the time the registrar leaves. Registrars will normally be booked at 20- or 30-minute intervals during the induction period, whereas the trainer will normally be seeing a patient every 10 minutes. It is helpful, therefore, for trainers to be booked at a lesser rate, with additional protected time at the end of the surgery when the registrar is first consulting. This allows the many questions that arise to be answered, either at the time or at the end of the surgery.

A slow, well-planned induction period enables a registrar to feel supported, to start to feel part of the primary care team and to understand the training process that is guiding him or her towards independent practice in a highly complex speciality. Habits learnt early in the induction period are difficult to break and they therefore need to be of a kind which is going to be helpful in the future.

The culture change from hospital to general practice can be destabilising and the quality of the induction and the time devoted to it can be the key to negotiating this transition successfully. General practice really does seem like the 'swampy ground' described by Schon,[16] where there are few right answers and, where answers exist, patients may choose not to follow them. Misselbrook's book, *Thinking about Patients*[17] also sheds light on why general practice can seem so daunting but also beautifully captures its challenge.

The induction process

The structure of the induction is the skeleton on which the process rests. Establishing an honest, trusting relationship between trainers and registrars is an important task in the induction period. Protected time for the tutorial each week allows trainers to help registrars to explore and define their educational needs. These can be very different from registrar to registrar, according to their background. Someone who has spent many years as a specialist registrar in obstetrics, and has perhaps done six months' paediatrics and six months' medicine will have different needs from a doctor who has gone straight from house jobs to a broadly based vocational training scheme with some experience already based in the community.

When assessing educational needs the curriculum vitae is the obvious place to start, but other tools such as confidence rating scales and phased evaluation programmes are also helpful. Examples of assessment tools can be found on most deanery websites (*see* www.londondeanery.ac.uk).

One of the main tasks of the early tutorials is to draw up a list of educational objectives that can be summarised in a personal development plan (PDP). This can then form the basis for an educational contract, signed by both parties, sent with the employment contract to the deanery. Although priorities may change as the year progresses, it is confidence-building for both registrar and trainer to see learning outcomes achieved.

The skills of trainers are tested in the early induction weeks when negotiating the shape of the PDP so that the ownership rests firmly with the registrar. The preferred learning style of both the learner and the teacher will become clearer during this process. If the match is similar, for instance if both learn most comfortably as 'activists'[18] then learning from patient encounters is ideal. However, if one or other of the pair is predominantly a 'theorist' then the activist may not understand why the tutorials are not perceived as being as useful as they might be.

During the induction period it is important to negotiate the content of the tutorial and who is going to lead the learning. Trainers may need to encourage registrars to become more active both in deciding *what* needs to be learnt and *how* this is going to occur as the coaching or educational facilitator style of one-to-one teaching can be both novel and threatening. In the early induction period registrars also need to be encouraged to keep a learning log, consisting of questions as they arise. Some of these will be simple to answer, such as 'How do I write a medical certificate?'. Others may be much more difficult, such as 'I know how to write a medical certificate but what do I do when I think the patient who is asking for a certificate has not really got backache?'.

Another important task in the first month is to help registrars to map out the normal timings for completing the various components of summative assessment and the MRCGP examination. Summative assessment may be enough for some registrars but, increasingly, where parts of the MRCGP examination are recognised for summative assessment purposes, registrars are keen to follow this route. Again, trainers need to be supportive in the induction period and give a sense of what is entailed to reach the required standard, what the assessment processes consists of and what can realistically be achieved in the time available.

Salaried and freelance GPs

This group includes locums, retainees, Flexible Career Scheme (FCS) doctors and returners, who all need an induction similar to the registrar's but modified according to their specific needs. They need to know how to use the computer system, what codes are used and what protocols are followed. Sitting in with other members of the team may be the best way of demonstrating the role of each primary care team member, and the context in which their work is carried out so the doctor will refer to that team member appropriately. It is also helpful to have a named person for a locum to turn to with queries. However, the induction by necessity will need to be shorter with the emphasis on meeting the team, learning about practice systems and referral patterns. Beware of skimping the induction: if it is too short neither the practice nor the locum will gain from the experience of working in the practice.

Returners, retainees and FCS doctors have mentoring time built into their week and have a named educational supervisor. They will need a similar induction to a registrar but modified appropriately, as they will have completed vocational training successfully and can work independently. Returners may have not worked for many years and may lack confidence so their induction will need to be carefully and slowly worked through with enough time for supervision built in.

Retainees and FCS doctors are those who, because of other commitments, cannot work full time. The role of the mentor is to facilitate the continuing professional development so that FCS doctors can successfully complete their yearly appraisal.

An induction pack for practices includes protocols, referral guides, etc, and is worth the time and energy spent in its creation, especially as written material is of proven worth.[6] However, because things change so fast someone needs to be in charge of keeping the pack updated. Locums may only work in the practice for a short period, but their induction is equally important and a good practice induction pack is invaluable for them. Personal medical services (PMS) doctors or partners joining a practice also deserve the same carefully thought out induction.

EU doctors entering general practice

EU doctors come to the UK as experienced doctors with considerable skills. Their induction relates more to getting used to a different healthcare system and a different medical and social culture rather than filling in gaps in clinical knowledge and experience. A 10-week induction programme introducing French doctors to the UK has been in operation in south-east London for the last three years.[19] The doctors spend half the week in a peer group with input from a skilled facilitator and half the week in a GP practice where they are introduced to the English system of seeing patients, recording consultations, referral systems, etc. As with EU hospital doctors help with language skills, especially medical English, is most appreciated. The key objectives for the programme were informed by the findings of a six-month induction programme for Soviet Union doctors settling in Israel.[20] Interestingly, this research showed these doctors might require more than three years of continuing support.

Refugee doctors

Refugee doctors often have considerable skills to offer their adopted country, but not only do they come with cultural differences they are usually also survivors of very traumatic events. Their experience of healthcare in their countries of origin will also be very different from the NHS. Because general practice is not the normal way of providing care in the countries that these doctors have come from, the GP London Deanery has developed a clinical attachment scheme which gives refugee doctors an experience of general practice as well as providing help with writing curriculum vitae and improving their English. This scheme has successfully enabled some doctors to train for general practice by entering mainstream vocational training schemes, and has allowed others to join the specifically created refugee vocational training schemes now established in north London. The overall principles of induction have been applied in the attachment schemes. Giving the doctor a sense of safety and self-esteem as described in Maslow's hierarchy of needs[21] may be as important as the induction provided.

Summary

The main aim of induction programmes for doctors in primary and secondary care, and at different training grades, is to assist them to settle quickly and efficiently into their new jobs. This, in turn, benefits patients, which is the main focus of every posting.

Careful planning, skilled support and staged written materials are themes that are common to all induction programmes. Several specific topics have also been raised that are specific to the particular training grade, the primary and secondary care setting of the posts and for doctors who have not trained in the UK or are returning to medicine after many years away from practice. Evaluation of different programmes has been positive for both participants and organisers. Such induction procedures play an important part in educational activities for all NHS doctors.

References

1 Standing Committee on Postgraduate Medical and Dental Education (1993) *A Good Start. A Report on Job Induction for Hospital Doctors and Dentists in Training.* SCOPE, London.

2 Paice E, Aitken M, Cowan G *et al.* (2000) Trainee satisfaction before and after the Calman reforms of specialist training: questionnaire survey. *BMJ.* **320**: 832–6.

3 Welsh C (2000) Training overseas doctors in the United Kingdom. They must be given accurate information about their job prospects. *BMJ.* **321**: 253–4.

4 Luck C (2000) Career focus: reducing stress among junior doctors. *BMJ.* **321**: 2.

5 Paice E and West G (1995) Senior House Officers: are overseas graduates treated differently? *British Journal of Hospital Medicine.* **53**: 203–6.

6 Ward SJ and Stanley P (1999) Induction for senior house officers. Part II: The departmental programme. *Postgraduate Med J.* **75**: 401–4.

7 Mitchell HE and Laidlaw JM (1999) Make induction day more effective – add a few problems. *Med Educ.* **33**: 424–8.

8 Ward SJ and Stanley P (1999) Induction for senior house officers. Part I The hospital programme. *Postgraduate Med J.* **75**: 346–50.

9 Gayed NM (1991) Residency directors' assessments of which selection criteria best predicted the performance of foreign-born foreign medical graduates during internal medicine residencies. *Acad Med.* **66**: 699–701.

10 Ewing H (1999) Induction down under. *Hospital Medicine.* **60**: 440–1.

11 Andrew R and Bates J (2000) Program for licensure for international medical graduates in British Columbia: 7 years experience. *CMAJ.* **162**: 801–3.

12 Ong YL, McFadden G and Gayen A (2000) Induction for overseas qualified doctors. *Hospital Medicine.* **63**: 558–60.

13 Ong YL and MacFadden G (2003) Inducting doctors from the European Union into the NHS. *BMJ: Careers Supplement.* 27/9. S99.

14 Ong YL, Gayen A (2003) Helping refugee doctors get their first jobs: the pan-London clinical attachment scheme. *Hospital Medicine.* **64**: 488–90.

15 Joint Committee on Postgraduate Training for General Practice (2001) *The Selection and Re-selection of GP Trainers.* JCPTGP, London.

16 Schon DA (1987) *Educating the Reflectice Practitioner.* Jossey-Bass, San Fransisco.

17 Misslebrook D (2001) *Thinking about Patients.* Pretoc Press, Newbury.

18 Honey P and Mumford A (1992) *The Manual of Learning Styles* (3e), (*See also* the Learning Styles Questionnaire: www.peterhoney.com).

19 Ballard KD and Laurence PB (2004) An induction programme for European general practitioners coming to work in England: development and evaluation. *Education in Primary Care.* **15**(4): 584–95.

20 Bernstein JH and Shuval JT (1998) The occupational integration of former Soviet physicians in Israel. *Soc Sci Med.* **47**: 809–19.

21 Maslow A and Lowery R (eds) (1998) *Towards a Psychology of Being* (3e). Wiley & Sons, New York.

CHAPTER 7

Career counselling

Colin Stern and Anthea Lints

The problem

The ultimate decision in selecting a medical career pathway is one that, in the UK, is left to the individual doctor. However, information to enlighten that choice is available to those who know how to access these resources and, just as we all have learning style preferences, the format in which information is available, be it one-to-one counselling, electronically accessed or the written word, should suit all tastes. Medicine offers many career possibilities which demand a variety of skills, but the profession has been slow to provide appropriate information to doctors in training about the skills and aptitudes they require. As a result, medical students and doctors in training use a variety of methods to help them settle on a final career. Their choices are not always best suited to the skills and aptitudes they possess.

A consequence of the mismatch between aspirations and opportunities is that many doctors waste time in their first few postgraduate years, trying to enter a speciality for which they are either not suited or insufficiently endowed with the attributes being sought.[1] Eleven years later, only 65% of doctors ended up in the speciality that was their first choice as pre-registration house officers (PRHOs).[2] Unavoidable limitations in the breadth of medical school curricula mean that there are many specialities that undergraduates never experience. Only a few medical schools have introduced a career counselling service for students which gives them the opportunity to experiment and explore during electives, along the lines of the model offered for the last 10 years by the Career Advisory Service of the American Association of Medical Colleges.

The National Health Service (NHS) is facing a crisis in primary care because of a looming shortage of general practitioners (GPs). Lambert and colleagues have shown how seldom general practice had been included in the initial selection of long-term careers.[3] It is a source of concern that less than 40% of doctors had considered this to be a career option on leaving medical school, when the NHS needs 50% of medical school output to go into general practice. A study of 100 pre-registration house officers (PRHOs) in London recently found that the number opting for general practice fell from 24% after six months to 18% at the end of their PRHO year. This finding, however, is not necessarily the case in all medical schools. It may partly be a consequence of the minimal interaction that GPs have with doctors in training and it may be that students are not able to appreciate the attractions of such a career so early.[4] Those who did consider a career in general practice at that stage tended to retain it as their chosen speciality. However, it is not unusual for doctors unhappy with their first-chosen speciality to retrain in general practice, a career change that is made more attractive by the willingness of the statutory body responsible for certification, the Joint Committee for Postgraduate Training in General Practice (JCPTGP), to consider experience acquired in other core specialities towards GP training.

The UK Medical Careers Group, based at the Institute of Health Sciences at the University of Oxford, has been carrying out detailed surveys on the careers of all UK medical graduates since 1995 and generating valuable information on the posts and pathways that they follow. If the improvements in medical training and education are matched by more appropriate and supportive career advice, it will be possible to track the way in which they affect the achievement of career posts.

Existing career advice arrangements

The career advice that students are offered at medical school is idiosyncratic. Although some schools offer one-to-one counselling, others run comprehensive careers fairs and a few provide a couple of lectures about medical specialities. New styles of medical school curricula provide more experience in primary care and some, such as Norwich, base their programme primarily in the community. Despite these welcome changes, most students receive the bulk of their learning in secondary and tertiary care environments and their career choices are influenced by these experiences.

There is no formal link between medical school careers advice and the service offered to PRHOs. Some medical schools recommend that their graduates should return to meet their student advisers, but most PRHOs rely on colleagues and consultants to shape their choices. At some trusts, the clinical tutor provides a career counselling service and there are a few trusts where this is an 'opt-out' session. However, the majority of PRHOs do not take the opportunity to discuss the appropriacy of their career aspirations. Course organisers responsible for general practice vocational training schemes (GPVTS) are willing to counsel those interested in general practice. Appraisal, which now underpins both basic speciality training (BST) and GPVTS, also provides an opportunity to discuss career progression. These arrangements are usually ad hoc and often rely on the initiative being taken by the junior doctor. It is anticipated that the foundation programmes that will be introduced to all graduates from medical schools in 2005 will have a much heavier emphasis on career advice, which is welcome.

Once a trainee enters higher speciality training the Speciality Training Committee (STC) and its officers begin to collect evidence of trainees' performance in a co-ordinated way. The Educational Superviser and the Programme Director are able to advise trainees about subspeciality aptitude in an informed fashion and continued conversations over the years of higher speciality training help to direct them into appropriate career posts. As a consequence of the poor career advice support that specialist registrars (SpRs) have received earlier in training, some are deemed unsuitable for their chosen speciality and compelled to change path. In-programme support is available in general practice for those on organised GPVTS. For those constructing their own programmes, the regulations can seem complicated and daunting. Advice is available from the JCPTGP, which publishes an excellent pamphlet entitled *A Guide to Certification*, which describes the various pathways to certification in depth.

Recently, the *British Medical Journal* (BMJ) has developed a career advice service. This is largely information-based, but offers a personal service for those that seek it. It is a valuable initiative, but it remains to be seen how effective it will be. The London Deanery has developed a web page[5] that provides detailed information about each of the medical and surgical specialities, and other deaneries have published handbooks on medical careers. As a result of these initiatives, there is plenty of information available to trainees. What was needed was better co-ordination of this information and a career advice programme which was based on a personal approach for each young doctor. The BMJ career service is co-ordinating access to the information available.

How trainee doctors make choices

PRHOs make their career decisions mostly by a process of exclusion,[3] and making choices is a combination of ruling some things in and others out. A few fall in love with a speciality at first sight and never seriously consider another, but most consider a wide range of options and discard them one by one in a process that has been likened to hypothesis generation and testing.[6]

PRHOs often feel confused and anxious about the career choices before them, and they need more support. In a large survey of PRHOs, less than a third were satisfied with the careers information provided by their consultant supervisor.[7] Career choices seem to be based on positive and negative experiences as students, the opinions of their peers and immediate seniors, and by their perceptions of the quality of life of those in the speciality. Broadly, lifestyle issues mould their views. Heavy on-call duties and hours of work, long training time and fear of litigation figure strongly as factors putting them off certain specialities. The competitiveness of a speciality is another feature.

A recent study showed that career choice by the majority of PRHOs becomes clearly defined during the second half of the PRHO year. However, those who were uncertain and then made their minds up were more likely to aspire to careers in hospital medicine than in primary care. In terms of workforce need, trainees seriously underestimated the likelihood of ultimately having a career in general practice. To a lesser extent, there were too few trainees seeking careers in pathology, psychiatry, imaging, and obstetrics and gynaecology. By the end of their post, 51% of PRHOs said that the greatest influence on their career choice had been their personal experiences, both positive and negative. When experience at medical school was added, this rose to 66%. By the end of post, PRHOs did not feel that they needed more advice, but were confident that they could manage their careers effectively.

Career advice tools and methods

There are sophisticated and validated tools and methods that have been widely used to support career counselling in fields outside medicine. A key factor in effective counselling has been shown to be the personality type of the subject. It has been shown that the way doctors in training cope with their learning environments is closely related to their personality type, and there is evidence that particular specialities of medicine tend to attract those with specific personality types.[8] Some suggest that it would be sensible for personal characteristics to be understood early: to enable learning to take place more effectively; to support students better; and to help guide trainees into careers that seem to suit them best. The Myers–Briggs Personality Profile has been widely used in this context and studies of medical graduates show a stable relationship between Myers–Briggs personality type and choice of speciality at residency matching.[9]

Gale and Grant[10] designed a computer programme, Sci45, based upon 130 structured questions about the working and lifestyle preferences of doctors in different specialities. Answering these questions allows the programme to recommend the 10 specialities to which the respondent seems best suited, as well as the 10 to which they seems least suited. A study has shown that although all PRHOs were eager to try the programme only a few found it useful. However, trainees who are completely at a loss in selecting a career path found Sci45 helpful in suggesting practical choices. It might prove helpful to have more instruments of this sort, perhaps measuring manual dexterity, pattern recognition or tolerance of ambiguity.

Many students have a limited perspective of the kaleidoscope of career opportunities that medicine has to offer. The *British Medical Journal* (BMJ) career advice initiative, coupled with the career fairs that the British Medical Association (BMA) offers, is helping to fill that gap. There are a variety of books, guides and websites that trainees can access. Some, such as the London Deanery website,[7] cover all possibilities and are regional; others, such as those established by the royal colleges, focused on a particular group of specialities.

However much information is made available, it will have a small influence upon career choice unless it is linked to a formal career advice structure through which every trainee passes. This structure must include sessions of one-to-one counselling with someone trained in career counselling, because students and trainees need individual support in order to talk through their aspirations and to set them against their potential. Not every trainee can become a professor of neurosurgery and realism needs to be injected sensitively into the discussion.

A suggested plan for the future

Improving the quality of career information, advice and counselling must become an important factor if the reforms of postgraduate medical training embodied in the 'Modernising Medical Careers' (MMC) initiative and leading into speciality training programmes are to be successful. Career development should be a continuous process, beginning in medical school. The personality of the student should be taken into account, both during undergraduate education and in considering the suitability of various career options. Some surgeons are convinced that they can identify a personality type associated with success in their field.[11] From a more individual point of view, quality of life has become increasingly important to young doctors when making their choices.

At medical school

Personality profiles derived for students on medical school entry may help to inform their individual learning and eventually to help with career choice. Continuity needs to be established between the advice provided by medical schools and that available for doctors in training. Initially, a dialogue between the postgraduate deanery and the medical schools should be established, with the objective of agreeing a joint process of career advice and counselling. The deaneries and the medical schools should share career counselling resources

A careers folder should be opened during the undergraduate course, to include all the information relevant to that student. This folder would be a discrete part of the documentation that trainees carry with them through to their career post appointment, together with their validation folder.

Foundation programmes

On graduation, doctors entering the new foundation programmes will need to build on the career planning carried out at medical school. The introduction of the foundation course will require a clearer knowledge of the balance between the aspirations of young doctors in training, their skills and attributes and the feasibility of pursuing their career choice. Ideally, the posts included in the programme will give doctors exposure, not only to specialities that they are considering but also to shortages in specialities that they may not have considered. Career counselling and support will be needed to help them identify the basic specialist training programme that matches most closely their aspirations and attributes.

All trusts need to ensure that every doctor in the first year of the foundation programme (FP1) meets the clinical tutor, or a suitable career adviser, early in the second six-month posting. This meeting should support the aspirations of the young doctor but, at the same time, should provide accurate information concerning the needs of the medical workforce and be realistic about the doctor's prospects in their chosen speciality. The information exchanged at this meeting should inform the choice of the second year of the foundation programme (FP2) selected by the trainee. FP2 programmes must deliver a wide variety of experiences and 'tasters', with as many as possible of them including a meaningful experience in primary care.

Basic specialist and higher specialist training

The pattern of basic specialist training (BST) is emerging. Programme training will be a paradigm of SpR training and will last between two and three years. Some programmes will be generic to begin with, but will offer opportunities for subspecialisation once the appropriate tests of ability and competence have been passed. Clearly, career advice will be integral to this process and should build upon the information already in the career folder. BST committees may need to designate a committee member to take primary responsibility for career advice to support education supervisors, who will inevitably be the port of first call to those seeking guidance.

As trainees progress into higher speciality training (HST) they will still need advice about research, out-of-programme experience, subspeciality options or what to do if they feel unsuited to their speciality. The STC already uses its knowledge of trainees to help in this work. More effective early support and advice should simplify the task and reduce the likelihood of a poor match between trainees and their chosen career path.

Conclusion

Career guidance ought to be offered early, based on evidence and tailored to the characteristics and needs of the individual. Every opportunity should be seized for young doctors to recognise the exciting possibilities open to them and to base their decisions on positive choice rather than an increasingly demoralising process of elimination. In order for this to happen we will need to develop career counsellors with the training, time and tools to do the job properly. Ideally, this will lead to a shared, nationally agreed process that is woven into the protocols that guide undergraduate and postgraduate medical education.

References

1 Paice E (2002) Career pathways. *BMJ*. **325**: S19.

2 Edwards C, Lambert TW, Goldacre MJ *et al.* (1997) Early medical career choices and eventual careers. *Med. Educ.* **31**: 237–42.

3 Lambert TW, Davidson JM, Evans J *et al.* (2003) Doctors' reasons for rejecting initial choice of specialities as long-term careers. *Med. Educ.* **37**: 312–18.

4 Blades DS, Ferguson G, Richardson HC *et al.* (2000) A study of junior doctors to investigate the factors that influence career decisions. *Br J Gen Prac*. **50**: 483–5.

5 www.londondeanery.ac.uk/CareerGuide/index.asp

6 Katz LA, Sarnacki RE and Schimpfhauser F (1984) The role of negative factors in changes in career selection by medical students. *Journal of Medical Education*. **59**: 285–90.

7 Gillard JH, Dent TH, Aarons EJ *et al.* (1993) Pre-registration house officers in eight English regions: survey of quality of training. *BMJ*. **307**: 1180–4.

8 Ferguson E, James D, O'Hehir F *et al.* (2003) Pilot study of personality, references and personal statements in relation to performance over five years of a medical degree. *BMJ*. **326**: 429–32.

9 Stillwell NA, Walick MM, Thal SE *et al.* (2000) Myers–Briggs type and medical speciality choice: a new look at an old question. *Teaching and Learning in Medicine*. **12**: 14–20.

10 Gale R and Grant J (2002) Sci45: the development of a speciality choice inventory. *Medical Education*. **36**: 659–66.

11 Thomas J (1997) The surgical personality: fact or fiction? *Am J Surg*. **174**: 573–7.

CHAPTER 8

Recruitment to specialist registrar and GP registrar training posts

Jane Appleyard, Anthea Lints and Neil Jackson

Introduction

The recruitment of doctors to the specialist and general practitioner (GP) training pathways quite rightly remains a high priority for the NHS, to ensure a quality medical workforce for patient care. This chapter will focus on the recruitment process and procedures for the specialist registrar (SpR) and GP registrar (GPR) grades. With patient safety a priority and the need to underpin this with professional competence, it becomes essential to select the best candidates for training by the most appropriate means.

Recruitment procedures and processes should encompass a number of core principles or characteristics, and the hallmarks of these are:

- validity
- reliability
- discriminating ability
- transparency
- feasibility
- legal defensibility.

In addition, equal opportunities and observance of employment law are essential.

Recruitment to specialist registrar training posts

Recruitment to the SpR grade for hospital medical and dental staff, and doctors in public health medicine is governed by the guidance provided by the

Department of Health, *A Guide to Specialist Registrar Training*,[1] which is usually referred to as the 'Orange Book'.

The guidance provided by the 'Orange Book' is in line with best practice as recommended by the Chartered Institute of Personnel and Development (CIPD) and complies with employment law, in particular in relation to anti-discrimination legislation. This chapter describes how the London Deanery has developed a recruitment methodology, that demonstrates transparency and equity to applicants and panel members alike.

Recruitment

The London Deanery is responsible for recruiting to the Specialist Registrar grade. This remit covers the following.

- The recruitment of SpRs to enter a training programme leading to the Certificate of Completion of Specialist Training (CCST), which is required for appointment to a consultant post. The training programmes usually last for five to six years and trainees appointed to an SpR programme will be awarded a national training number (NTN) or visiting training number (VTN), depending on their residency status. Applicants must meet the entry criteria laid down by the appropriate college or faculty.
- The recruitment of fixed-term training appointments, which offer structured training but do not lead to the CCST. These typically last for one to two years of training. Doctors appointed to fixed-term training appointments are usually overseas doctors who do not have right of residence. Applicants do not have to meet the entry criteria, but should have equivalent training and experience.
- The recruitment of locum appointments for training (LATs), which offer structured training but do not lead to the CCST. These appointments are usually between one and three years in duration, and time in a LAT post will count towards the CCST after appointment to an NTN or VTN. Applicants must meet the entry criteria laid down by the appropriate college or faculty.

Although recruitment activity will vary from year to year, the London Deanery averages about 150 recruitment campaigns a year, attracting about 5 000 applications and appointing over 1 000 trainees to SpR positions. The number of applicants applying for each campaign will vary by speciality and it is not uncommon for popular specialities to receive more than a 100 applications.

Recruitment planning

The London Deanery recommends that, wherever possible, recruitment is planned at least 12 months in advance of positions becoming available. The Chair of the Speciality Training Committee (STC) or the Training Programme Director (TPD) will look at the current stock of trainees and make an assessment of the number of vacancies needing to be filled at the next recruitment episode. This assessment will take into account any vacancies resulting from trainees completing the programme and obtaining the CCST, and any shorter term vacancies resulting from trainees taking time out of the training programme for research or some other out-of-programme experience or special leave, such as for maternity. The process also needs to take into account any trainees who are returning to the programme after an agreed period of absence.

As well as assessing the potential number of vacancies available, the Chair of the STC or the TPD will also need to decide what sort of training the speciality can offer. Where an SpR on the award of a CCST is releasing an NTN or a VTN, it will be possible to recruit a new entrant to the training programme. Where the vacancy to be covered is short-term, the post will be advertised either as a fixed-term training appointment or as an LAT.

In larger specialities, such as anaesthetics, an annual recruitment cycle can be agreed because of the large numbers completing the training programme each year. At regular intervals (every three to four months) throughout the year a recruitment episode is timetabled and information about the annual timetable is publicised on the London Deanery website.[2] The Chair of the STC or the TPD will review the current stock of trainees as each recruitment episode approaches. In smaller specialities it may be less easy for recruitment to be planned in advance and ad hoc episodes may have to be held. Wherever possible, the recruitment arrangements outlined below are adhered to.

Having assessed the likely number of vacancies and decided how these are to be filled, the next step is to decide when it would be appropriate to advertise. When making this decision account will be taken of the timing of any college or faculty examinations and the starting date of the post. Ideally, the timetable should allow for the appointments committee to meet three months before the vacancy is due to occur, to allow time for the successful applicant(s) to resign from their current posts.

The suggested minimum recruitment timetable is:

- advert appears: Week 1
- closing date: end of Week 3
- shortlisting committee: Week 4
- Interview committee: Week 6.

Where a speciality attracts large numbers of applicants, the timetable will be extended to allow additional time for processing applications. The panel membership is agreed at the same time as the timetable. Administrative support for the committee is furnished by the London Deanery and the constitution is laid down by the 'Orange Book' and consists of:

- a Lay Chair
- the regional college adviser or a nominated deputy
- the relevant postgraduate dean or a nominated deputy
- representatives of the consultant staff involved in the training programme (minimum of two and maximum of four)
- a nominee from the appropriate university
- the programme director or chair of the STC
- a representative of senior management in an employing trust in the training rotation.

Using this framework, the London Deanery will constitute a committee that comprises an appropriate balance between all interests. Because of the size of the SpR training programmes, it is not possible for all the consultant staff involved in the training programme to participate in the recruitment process, and the STC will agree which consultants should represent the wider body. Where the training programme involves trainees working in another deanery, representatives from that deanery will also be invited to sit on the panel. Every consultant who sits on a deanery appointment panel must have had equal opportunities or interview skills training. Consultants can obtain this training through their trust or through training courses run by the London Deanery.

Recruitment documentation

The London Deanery has developed structured recruitment paperwork that provides a framework by which applications can be assessed. The structured paperwork has been developed after a review of recruitment documentation at the time of the introduction of the SpR grade. The review was informed by the proceedings of five focus groups, which considered the characteristics of a successful consultant and identified 11 major competencies. These were further broken down by key characteristics, and the review made recommendations as to when and how these should be evaluated during the recruitment process. This work resulted in the development of generic recruitment paperwork, which has been adapted by each speciality.

The cornerstone of the structured documentation is the person specification. Based on the key characteristics identified in the review exercise, the generic specification is adapted by each speciality to reflect speciality-specific criteria, for example the entry criteria laid down by the college or faculty, including knowledge and skills. An example of part of a person specification for trauma and orthopaedic surgery is shown in Figure 8.1.

	Essential	When evaluated	Desirable	When evaluated
Qualifications	• Eligible for registration with the GMC	AF	• BSc (or other intercalated degree)	AF
	• MB BS (or equivalent)	AF	• Higher research degree in orthopaedic or other surgical speciality (e.g. PhD, MD, MS, MSc)	AF
	• MRCS/FRCS or equivalent	AF		
Clinical experience	• 12 months SHO post in trauma and orthopaedic surgery (or equivalent)	AF	• Experience in other related specialities (e.g. neurosurgery, plastic surgery, vascular surgery, cardiac surgery).	AF
	• 6 months SHO in A&E	AF	• Additional medical or orthopaedic experience (e.g. overseas)	AF
			• ATLS course	AF
			• ATLS instructor	AF

AF = application form

Figure 8.1

An application form was developed to reflect the competencies identified in the generic person specification. This was designed to enable shortlisters to formally assess candidates against specific areas of the person specification. The competencies that are identified in the person specification as being evaluated at the shortlisting stage are listed on the shortlisting score sheet. The shortlisting score sheet lists the entry criteria for the programme (as laid down by the appropriate royal college or faculty) and the essential and desirable criteria agreed by the STC. Shortlisters are required to work within a narrow scoring range of 0, 1 or 2, where 0 means that there is little or no evidence of the attribute being present, 1 means that the attribute is present and 2 means that the attribute is present 'in abundance'. Part of the shortlisting score sheet for trauma and orthopaedics is reproduced in Figure 8.2.

The recruitment paperwork also includes a score sheet, which panel members use to record the performance of candidates at interview. The interview score sheet, like the shortlisting score sheet is derived from the person specification. Panel members have space to record brief notes about the interview as well as scoring the candidates using the score range of 0, 1 or 2.

Both the shortlisting score sheet and the interview score sheet can be adapted to suit the particular requirements of the speciality. Using the framework of the person specification, attributes can be weighted to reflect speciality requirements. For example, a speciality that has a strong academic base might choose to expand the section of the score sheet relating to publications by awarding

Essential criteria	Maximum score (range 0–2)	Applicant's score	Assessed in this section of the application form
			C
12 months' experience in trauma and orthopaedic surgery	1		D, E & J
6 months SHO in A&E	1		D, E & J
			D, E & J
Procedures undertaken personally (e.g. DHS, hemi-arthroplasty, simple fracture fixation, day case surgery)	2		F

Figure 8.2

points for first author papers, points for abstracts and points for other publications, thus allowing a total of six points for this attribute.

The final document that forms part of the structured recruitment paperwork is the professional reference form. Again, this is derived from the person specification and its purpose is to comment on those characteristics that cannot be evaluated in any other way. The reference request form has been designed to ask for comments on these characteristics. Where a referee has a concern about an applicant's abilities, these should be described on the reference request form.

The paperwork that is sent to panel members includes training notes explaining the process and the scoring system. Panel members are also sent guidance on interviews and examples of criterion-based questions.

The application process

All appointments are advertised in the *British Medical Journal* and on the website www.doctors.net.uk. Posts are advertised with a closing date of at least two weeks after the insertion date. Applications may be obtained either by post, by email or by downloading the application form from the doctors.net website.

Applicants are sent, or may download, the application pack. This contains a covering letter that explains how the appointments process works, gives details of the closing, shortlisting and interview dates, contact information for the recruitment process and the details of any members of the STC or websites which are available to provide additional details. The pack also contains the speciality training prospectus and any other information relevant to the appointment. The training prospectus and additional information will also be available on the London Deanery website.[2] Applicants are sent a copy of the shortlisting score sheet for information and this can be used by candidates for self-assessment purposes.

Applicants who wish to train on a less than whole-time basis (flexible training) are not required to declare this at the application stage. Applicants who wish to undertake training on a flexible basis are advised to discuss their circumstances with the London Deanery before making an application so that if they are appointed, arrangements for flexible training can be implemented without unnecessary delay.

Because of the nature of the posts, applicants for SpR posts are required to complete a declaration regarding fitness to practise and criminal convictions. This declaration forms part of the application form. Applicants who respond positively on the declaration must include with their application a separate sheet that explains the reason for the positive declaration with any further details they may wish to supply. For the most part, positive declarations relate to minor traffic offences, but occasionally a more serious issue is brought to light and in such cases senior staff at the London Deanery consider the issue before the application is put forward for consideration by the shortlisting panel. Positive declarations relating to minor offences are not routinely disclosed to panel members. Where a more serious offence is declared, the London Deanery will advise the lay chair and the STC chair and discuss whether this should affect consideration of the candidate for shortlisting or interview.

Once the closing date is reached, the applications received are copied and sent out to panel members, together with shortlisting score sheets, against which panel members will assess the applications.

The shortlisting process

The London Deanery requires that a shortlisting panel forms part of each recruitment event. Unless otherwise agreed, it is expected that all members of the appointments panel attend the shortlisting panel. In specialities where the number of applications is low, the Deanery may agree that the shortlisting panel be held using a conference call facility.

The London Deanery recommends that panel members review the applications and complete the shortlisting score sheets before attending the committee meeting. Where a speciality receives a large number of applications, it is possible for panel members to be allocated sections of the application form to mark. This will be agreed before recruitment takes place and, where necessary, the documentation will be amended to reflect this arrangement.

At the start of the meeting the lay chair will confirm with the STC chair or the TPD the number of vacancies available, as additional vacancies may have arisen since the advertisement appeared. The panel will also be asked to decide on the approximate number of applicants which it is reasonable to shortlist. This will depend on the number of training placements identified. As a rule of thumb, one or two applicants should be shortlisted for each vacancy available. The panel will then consider the applications received.

As a first step, the lay chair will ask the panel if any of the applicants should not be considered because they do not fulfil the entry requirements or because they have scored a 0 for an essential criterion. These candidates are discussed and where candidates are eliminated from consideration at this stage, the reasons for so doing are recorded.

The scores of the remaining applicants are then sorted into score order and the results given to panel members. For preference the scores are displayed using an overhead projector, but if this facility is not available copies of the spreadsheet recording the scores and calculations will be made available to committee members.

The panel then needs to consider the candidates in score order. The lay chair will ask whether any panel member does not agree with the order as displayed on the spreadsheet. If it is felt that a candidate has achieved a higher or lower score than their application might warrant, the lay chair will lead a discussion, which will be recorded.

If there are no objections to the order of the candidates, the lay chair will then ask the panel to consider how many candidates should be called for interview. The earlier discussions will have identified the number of vacancies and the possible number of candidates who might be called for interview, but this will now be finalised on the basis of the scoring. The panel will agree the cut-off point by using the score recorded for the candidates. This may result in the final shortlist being longer or shorter than originally proposed if scores are close. The lay chair should ensure that all panel members are happy with the cut-off point.

Once a shortlist has been agreed, the lay chair will discuss with the panel the format of the interviews and agree the areas that each panel member will cover during questioning. The 'Orange Book' lays down the composition of the interview panel, but the format of the interviews is not specified. Where few candidates are being interviewed, a panel interview is the preferred format. Where more candidates are being interviewed, the panel may wish to be divided into two or more smaller panels. The panel may also wish to consider whether other assessment methods could be usefully employed. Obstetrics and gynaecology uses an objective structured clinical examination to evaluate candidate performance in dealing with giving patients bad news.

The interview process

Interview panels convene at least 30 minutes before the first candidate is scheduled. Before the interviews commence, the lay chair will confirm the final list of training positions that are available and the type of training on offer. Where there are a number of posts or programmes available the candidates attending for interview may be given a sheet listing the vacancies on which they can indicate their preference.

Panel members use the interview score sheet as a tool to assess candidates. The interview score sheet reflects the criteria listed on the person specification that are to be evaluated at interview and uses the close ranking system of 0, 1 or 2. The lay chair will discuss with panel members the questions that will be asked to assess the criteria on the interview score sheet. Where an attribute has been assessed at the shortlisting stage, the same ground should not be covered again unless there is a need to elucidate or expand the information already obtained. Candidates are interviewed for a minimum of 30 minutes.

The lay chair and the STC chair will read the references before the interview to identify if any areas of concern exist. If the references do highlight concerns on the part of the referee, these should be explored with the candidate as part of the interview process.

When all candidates have been interviewed and scored, the scores from panel members are entered onto the interview score spreadsheet. This calculates the total interview score for each applicant and calculates a final score, which includes a percentage that represents the shortlisting score (usually 30% shortlist and 70% interview). The candidates are ranked in score order and presented to the panel. The panel will then discuss the ranking of the candidates and agree which candidates should be offered appointments. The panel will also agree whether any applicants are deemed unappointable and consider the arrangements for feedback to unsuccessful applicants. The recruiting agent will record the decisions of the panel.

Where candidates have been invited to wait or to return for the result of the interview, successful candidates will be invited back to meet the panel so that the appointment may be confirmed. The lay chair is responsible for advising the successful candidates of:

- the type of appointment offered (NTN/VTN, FTTA, LAT)
- the location of the initial placement (if known)
- the year of entry into the programme
- the duration of the contract for the initial placement.

Candidates who wish to train flexibly will advise the committee of their wishes at this point. The panel will then need to consider how flexible training can be accommodated within the training programme either by job share or a reduced session commitment. Because those training flexibly will take longer to complete the training, an additional NTN may be granted to appoint a full-time SpR.

Some candidates may wish to defer entry into the training programme because of research commitments. Where the research commitment is for a period of two years or more, the lead dean may grant an additional NTN to allow the substantive post to be filled.

Occasionally an unexpected vacancy can occur in the period immediately following a recruitment episode. Where this occurs, the STC chair will decide whether a new recruitment episode should be undertaken or whether any candidates who were interviewed in the previous round should be considered for the vacancy.

Following the interview panel

After the interview panel has met and selected candidates for appointment, the offers of appointment must be confirmed in writing and trusts informed of the names of new joiners to the programme. The paperwork from the panel meetings, including the scoresheets and notes made by panel members are stored for 12 months by the London Deanery. The recruitment paperwork and process will be reviewed, if appropriate, before the next round of recruitment.

Recruitment to general practice training posts

Since 2000, recruitment to general practice training posts has been channelled through a centralised process, organised by deaneries and co-ordinated by the National Recruitment Office (NRO) following guidance provided by the Department of Health in *The GP Registrar Scheme – Vocational Training for General Medical Practice – the UK Guide*,[3] which is usually referred to as the 'Green Book'. Most deaneries recruit twice yearly. The crucial dates are advertised on the NRO website (www.gprecruitment.org.uk). The recruitment process has been designed to comply with equal opportunities legislation and employment law, and all training posts are subject to open competition. There are many similarities, therefore, with recruitment to SpR training posts as described earlier. Here, reference is made specifically to the differences in the process and the information given refers exclusively to recruitment to general practice training posts.

General practice training

Normally general practice training consists of 24 months in a variety of educationally approved senior house officer (SHO) posts followed by 12 months as a general practice registrar (GPR) in an approved training practice. The statutory organisation that oversees training and which, when training is completed, will issue a Certificate of Satisfactory Completion of Training (CSCT) is the Joint Committee for Postgraduate Training in General Practice (JCPTGP). The JCPTGP considers variations on the normal components of training, for example experience acquired abroad or experience in specialities not included in the core specialities. Core specialities are accident and emergency, care of the elderly, general medicine, obstetrics and gynaecology, paediatrics and psychiatry, and it is expected that a doctor training for a career in general practice will have experience in at least two of these. The regulations allow a considerable amount of flexibility in fulfilling the requirements of the 'middle year', which allow for diversity of experience, the introduction of innovative training posts and acknowledges the many routes to general practice. The regulations are described in greater detail in a pamphlet written by the JCPTGP, *A Guide to Certification*.[4] Training can therefore be acquired in several ways and a variety of training opportunities is available. Most deaneries offer the 'complete package' – a three-year GP vocational training scheme that entirely satisfies the statutory requirements. For doctors who have already completed one or two approved SHO posts, or who are changing career, or who come with some experience from abroad, there are shortened GP vocational training schemes and for those whose hospital experience satisfies the JCPTGP regulations, there are 12-month GPR posts. Entering a training programme will normally (provided progress is satisfactory) culminate in a JCPTGP certificate entitling the holder to work unrestrictedly as a GP performer in the NHS or within the EU. This is comparable with a CCST for hospital consultants. Those appointed to a GP training post will be given a National Training Number (NTN) by the appointing deanery.

The role of the National Recruitment Office

The NRO works on behalf of all deaneries in England, and reports directly to the Committee of GP Education Directors (COGPED). Wales, Scotland and Northern Ireland have separate arrangements. The NRO is supported by a national recruitment steering group and three subgroups, which cover issues of probity, procedures and process. The intention is to develop a standardised national approach to recruitment for general practice across all deaneries, which will be performance-managed through the NRO.

Adverts inviting applications for GP training posts appear in the BMJ, usually in January and July, for posts starting at least six months later. Precise instructions appear in the advert on how to download application forms and relevant information guiding applicants through the process. The NRO website includes a great deal of invaluable information, including the answers to frequently asked questions (FAQs) and details of eligibility for training posts. Those applying for shortened schemes or for 12-month GPR posts must ensure that their previous experience has been formally accepted by the JCPTGP, and as this can take some time (with supporting evidence required before a decision can be reached), candidates are well-advised to have this arranged in good time. This is especially true of experience acquired abroad. Otherwise, VTR2 certificates, usually provided by medical staffing departments at trust hospitals or downloaded from the JCPTGP website (www.jcptgp.org.uk), will be required as evidence by deaneries of satisfactory completion of SHO posts that applicants have done independently.

Like SpR posts, the number of vacancies varies depending on a number of factors, not least the availability of funding for education and training. The London Deanery website[2] gives approximate numbers of vacancies for that recruitment round. These numbers can be inaccurate because the invitation to apply is advertised eight months before posts start and funding and availability can vary during this time.

Each deanery has its own application form (based on a national template), and variations in methods of selection (which are currently being evaluated as we work towards a standardised approach across deaneries). In the London Deanery the recruitment and selection process is described in an eponymous document.[5] The application form contains demographic details and a series of short essay-type questions. These are designed to explore the mandatory and desirable criteria, which are described within the application pack outlining the characteristics sought. This is comparable with the person specification described earlier in this chapter. The competencies identified in the generic person specification are reflected in the application form and are used in the assessment of candidates at shortlisting and interview. These competencies were agreed after national consultation and consensus of the attributes of a successful GP. Curriculum vitae are not required. In addition to each deanery's unique application form, other standardised information is required by recruitment departments, for example equal opportunities and disability monitoring forms, a declaration regarding fitness to practise and criminal convictions, and references. It is the applicant's responsibility to ensure that three references are received by the deanery in good time. Because of the volume of applications received, incomplete applications are not considered so it is prudent that applicants follow the instructions to the letter. The closing date is precisely that and no application received after that date will be considered. Applicants are advised to include a stamped self-addressed envelope if they require confirmation that their application has been received. Although there is a national shortage of GPs, there is currently no shortage of applicants applying for a very limited number of training places. In London, every six months, we can expect more than 1 000 applications for approximately 200 training posts.

The shortlisting process

In the London Deanery, every completed application form that is eligible for the post applied for will be sent to three experienced, trained panel members for shortlisting. Applicants who do not fulfil all mandatory criteria will not be considered for interview. The essential attributes sought are as follows:

- clear and appropriate written communication skills
- a sense of empathy and understanding
- certain personal attributes, such as initiative, drive and enthusiasm
- an ability to cope with pressure
- organisation and delegation skills
- an appreciation of teamwork
- a commitment to learning and professional development.

Where there is disagreement between panel members, the application will be discussed formally by panel members until a consensus is reached.

The interview process

A limited number of applicants will be invited to interview, depending upon the number of training places available. In London, the interview panel consists of three experienced trainers, course organisers or hospital consultants, all of whom have attended equal opportunities and interview skills training. Questions at interview will explore the following areas:

- clinical knowledge and expertise
- communication skills
- empathy and understanding
- personal attributes
- coping with pressure
- integrity
- administrative skills
- teamwork.

Training posts will be allocated on performance at interview. Unlike the method used for SpR posts, the shortlisting score is not considered at this point, except when two candidates have the same score and only one post is available. Offers of training places will be made formally, shortly after interview but successful candidates are under no obligation to accept an offer until a specific date. Entry may not be deferred. Those not offered a post may be eligible for local or national clearing. Unsuccessful applicants may request written feedback so that subsequent applications can be made with understanding of problems and insight. Lately, however, it is the mismatch between huge numbers of suitable candidates and the paucity of available training posts rather than deficiencies in candidates' performances which have led to excellent candidates being denied training posts.

Allocation of posts

The specific composition of three-year rotations offered will be at the discretion of the course organiser responsible for the particular vocational training scheme. Shortened schemes, comprising one or two SHO posts and a GPR post, will be allocated centrally depending on ranking, availability of posts and the particular needs of the successful candidate. Twelve-month GPR posts are allocated locally by individual trainers' group co-ordinators in line with local agreements.

The comments above refer specifically to the process of recruitment adopted by the London Deanery – other deaneries have developed other methods of selection and, as time and experience build up, it is possible that a national process will evolve.

Tips and pitfalls

- Consult the NRO website and be certain you are eligible for the sort of training programme for which you are applying.
- If you are applying for a shortened GP vocational training scheme or a GPR post, ensure that your previous experience has been formally approved by the JCPTGP – failure to do so will delay your application.
- If you are completing SHO posts that are educationally approved for GP training, and have independently constructed your own hospital experience, be sure that you have collected and had endorsed VTR2 forms for each post before applying for a GPR post. Deaneries will want evidence that these posts are suitable and have been completed to a satisfactory standard before considering you for a GPR post.
- Read the application pack carefully – the characteristics sought are explicit and can mean the difference between success and failure.
- Where you are asked to make one choice – do not tick all the boxes (three-year GP vocational training scheme, shortened GP vocational training scheme, GPR post). You will only be invited to one interview and that will be for a specific sort of training post.
- Answer the essay-type questions succinctly, using personal experience to illustrate the characteristics sought. Limit your answers to the word count requested.
- Do not collaborate – the answers must be your own. Plagiarism will not be tolerated.
- Make sure that your application reaches its destination in good time and not at the last hour of the closing date. Confirm that the recruitment administrators have received your application by whatever means that particular deanery suggests.
- You are responsible for your references being received by the recruitment office.
- If you are invited for interview, make sure you arrive at the correct venue, on the right day and in good time.
- Prepare for interview with a 'dry run'. The areas to be explored are well advertised; normally, questions will explore your previous behaviour in certain circumstances so rehearse examples that might be reasonably anticipated to appear.
- Try not to discuss the interview with other applicants – on one occasion an applicant did just that, oblivious to the fact that the applicant he interrogated had been interviewed by a different panel. He was not appointed, as his answers seemed to bear no relationship to the questions asked.

The process can appear confusing and complicated, but this relatively new centralisation of recruitment underpinned by the work of the NRO has ensured a fairer, more transparent system.

Further information

- Department of Health (1998) *The Recruitment of Doctors and Dentists in Training.* DoH, London.(www.dh.gov.uk/PublicationsAndStatistics/LettersAndCirculars/ HealthServiceCirculars/HealthServiceCircularsArticle/fs/en?CONTENT_ID= 4004402&chk=sIWM13)

- Department of Health (2002) *Pre and Post Employment Checks for Doctors in England and Wales* (HSC/2002/008). DoH, London. (www.dh.gov.uk/PublicationsAndStatistics/LettersAnd Circulars/HealthServiceCirculars/HealthServiceCircularsArticle/fs/en?CONTENT_ID= 4004999&chk=JPAvUT)

- London Deanery (2002) *Recruitment to London/Essex and Herts/Kent, Surrey and Sussex (KSS) Specialist Registrar Training Programmes.* London Deanery, London.

- London Deanery (2002) I*nformation Pack for Associate Deans and Specialty Training Committees.* London Deanery, London.

References

1   Department of Health (1998) *A Guide to Specialist Registrar Training.* (the 'Orange Book'.) DoH, London. (www.publications.doh.gov.uk/medicaltrainingintheuk/orangebook.htm)

2   www.londondeanery.ac.uk

3   Department of Health (2000) *The GP Registrar Scheme – Vocational Training for General Medical Practice – the UK Guide.* (The 'Green Book'.) DoH, London.

4   Joint Committee on Postgraduate Training for General Practice (2002) *A Guide to Certification.* JCPTGP, London.

5   London Deanery (2003) *Recruitment Handbook – A Guide to Recruiting and Selecting Specialist Registrars.* London Deanery, London.

CHAPTER 9

Educating doctors for diversity

Antony Americano

Introduction

Equalities and diversity became firm fixtures on the medical and dental education agenda more than 20 years ago. Growing concerns about social inclusion, published research and a developing framework of equalities-focused legislation have maintained this position through the years.

The National Health Service (NHS) as an organisation has embraced these complex issues. A range of initiatives have had at their core the objective of increasing access to healthcare for all and ensuring that this care is provided by a workforce that is representative of the population it serves. Nevertheless, tensions are possible when these objectives are balanced with the need to develop a workforce fit for purpose in order to provide high-quality and safe patient care. Understood carefully, these tensions can be managed, reduced and even turned into positive experiences for those involved.

This chapter explores the equalities and diversity framework within which postgraduate medical and dental education operates. It will also analyse statistics on the trainee medical workforce. It will show that this is a time of significant demographic change in the workforce, and that real concerns exist about discrimination in medicine. The chapter proposes that an effective response in medical education involves mainstreaming equalities and diversity in both training and service delivery.

Defining the terms

The difference between equalities and diversity can be confusing. For some, the concept of diversity is an old idea dressed up in new clothes. Indeed, diversity does encompass the traditional equalities approach, with its focus on social concerns about imbalance in relation to specific groups protected by legislation. However, diversity also adds to this approach by encouraging a wider understanding of difference, both visible and invisible.[1] This is well conceptualised by Jehn *et al.*[2] who propose a three-factor model of diversity, as follows.

- Social category diversity concerns demographic differences, such as gender and ethnicity, which are core equal opportunities concerns in postgraduate medical and dental education and are discussed later on. Jehn *et al.*[2] theorised that difficulties in this factor would affect group communication and cohesion.
- Informational diversity (also known as 'organisational diversity') refers to diversity of background, such as knowledge, education, experience, tenure and function. Those from a medical and dental background are recognised as distinct 'tribes' among other 'tribes' such as nurses and other healthcare workers. Within the broad discipline of medicine there is a multitude of such distinctions, and it is thought that these differences also affect group communication and cohesion as well as generating higher task-related conflict.
- Value diversity (also known as 'psychological diversity') includes differences in personality and attitudes. A rich source of difference, but one that has the potential to affect individual, team and organisational life. This raises issues of 'team fit' and personality clashes as well as fundamentally different philosophical approaches to life. If this difference cannot be managed it can lead to conflict within teams, across professional groups and with patients and carers.

As diversity is a multidimensional concept, that is to say, individuals will belong to different factors across and between the concept, its study is complex. Each category will be a useful factor in understanding individuals but no single element will clearly define the unique nature of an individual.

It is perhaps no surprise that the literature studying the effect, positive or negative, of diversity on group performance and behaviour is generally inconclusive. Different studies show a complex range of results, which were hard to generalise because of the limitations of the studies themselves and the difficulty in controlling for variables. In addition, it is theorised that the value of diversity to group performance may depend on the type of task required of the group. The value may be particularly high when understanding a particular social category is a benefit, but the value will be less, or even non-existent, when tasks do not require such understanding.[3]

A framework for diversity

Diversity in postgraduate medical and dental education is best understood in context. A key influence is the standard expected of all doctors. The General Medical Council (GMC) publication, *Good Medical Practice*[4] states that doctors must not discriminate against colleagues because of their views on a range of factors, including their culture, beliefs, race or colour. Consequently, it is important that junior doctors are educated in this standard either through direct training or via modelling from senior colleagues. Formal learning is not always easy because trainees feel highly pressured to focus their development time on clinical competencies. Consequently, 'soft' skills and knowledge areas can be marginalised.

Another key influence is Government policy. Equality, fair treatment and social inclusion lie at the heart of Government plans to modernise the NHS. *The NHS Plan*[5] and *Shifting the Balance of Power*[6] acknowledge the diverse society in the UK and establish as core principles that the NHS will:

- shape services around the needs of patients
- support frontline staff to better respond to the needs of all sections of the community and deliver more responsive, high-quality services
- challenge discrimination on the grounds of age, gender, ethnicity, religion, disability and sexuality.

These principles are central to good clinical governance, to effective risk management and to attracting, retaining and developing the diverse workforce needed to fulfil the modernisation agenda.[7] As a consequence, the 'Positively Diverse' programme was developed in the NHS to encourage equality and diversity in the workplace.

Arguably the strongest framework for equalities is the law. There is an increasing body of legislation covering issues of discrimination, which is added to yearly by case law. As postgraduate medical and dental education works hard to address the established legislation on gender and racial discrimination, new challenges have arisen around human rights, disability, age, religion, gender reassignment and sexual orientation. A full discussion of these issues is beyond the scope of this chapter but is nevertheless worthy of further study in order to understand equalities.

One aspect of the law that will be covered, is the Race Relations (Amendment) Act 2000. This has placed a new and important statutory duty on public bodies to promote race relations. This applies to both the NHS and to higher education organisations covering the full gamut of the medical and dental student's experience. This requires, among other things, that:

- students from all ethnic backgrounds are equally satisfied with their education
- levels of educational achievement are high, with all students achieving their full potential
- the trainees are representative of the relevant population from which it recruits (NB the London Deanery has agreed with the Commission for Racial Equality (CRE) that this should be the population data for England)

- generally, the level of complaints is low, and there are no significant differences between ethnic groups in complaints about admission, training posts,
teaching, assessment and support.[8]

Evidence of compliance with this duty will include a demonstration of strong
leadership, one result of which will be that deanery staff and stakeholders are
trained in their responsibilities to promote race equality. Additionally, clear
policies are required as is assessment and publishing of results. This is all the
more complex for postgraduate medical and dental education where training is
carried out in a service environment, requires employment relationships with
trusts and is based on the involvement of Royal Colleges and a diverse range of
other bodies. It is also worth noting that though this legalisation only covers
race, other issues such as gender may be covered in the future and this is worth
bearing in mind when collecting data and planning training programmes.

The medical workforce – trainees and trainers

The frameworks identified above provide direction for managing equalities in
the trainee medical workforce. It is also important to consider this in the wider
educational context. Over more than a decade, there has been a considerable
expansion of student numbers in higher education. In the midst of this expansion, women have increased their representation from about a third in 1975 to
slightly more than half currently.[9] Nevertheless, despite gains in educational
qualifications, this success is not fully realised in the employment arena. Occupational gender stereotyping is still quite prevalent as exampled by nursing and
other professions allied to medicine, where women predominate. Do the same
barriers exist in medicine? This will be explored shortly.

Turning first to the issue of ethnicity, the percentage of young people in education who come from minority ethnic groups is significantly higher than for
white students. Amongst ethnic minority groups 81% of 16–19-year-olds were
in education and training and 42% of 20–24-year-olds. This compares with lower
figures for white students, among whom 67% of 16–19-year-olds were in education and training and 27% of 20–24-year-olds.[10] Of those entering higher
education whose ethnicity was known, 13% were from minority ethnic groups
who make up only 8% of the overall population. Of course, it is worth noting
that ethnic minorities generally have a lower mean age than the English population. Moving on to consider subjects, the most popular for home students from
ethnic minorities were pharmacy (37% of all students) and dentistry (35% of all
students). Pre-clinical medicine, which attracts in the region of 25% of students
from ethnic minorities, also scored highly particularly for students from an Asian
background.[11]

Do these demographic trends translate into changes in the medical workforce
and if so what are the implications? To consider this, it is necessary to look at

the available statistics. From the perspective of postgraduate medical and dental education this means looking at the trainees, registrars from a deanery perspective, and their trainers, who are in the main consultants or GPs. The focus will be on a review of figures for 1991 and 2000 for secondary care, and for 1990 and 2002 for primary care.

Table 9.1 looks at the ethnicity of secondary care registrars and consultants, and here comparisons between the 1991 and 2000 figures are complicated by the high level of 'Unknown' in the 1991 figures and the significant increase in registrar and consultant numbers between the two periods (by 23% and 45%, respectively). Inferences made from such data must therefore be treated with caution. In numerical terms, there is a large increase in the number of registrars and consultants from an ethnic minority, in particular from an Asian background. In percentage terms, the increase in registrars defining themselves as Asian (from 9% of the 1991 total to 23% of the 2000 total) suggests a meaningful increase in ethnic minorities among this group. This information is congruent with Higher Education Statistics Agency (HESA) data[11] indicating the popularity of medicine among students from an Asian background during this period.

Table 9.1: Comparison of ethnicity of registrars and consultants: 1991 and 2000

Ethnicity	1991				2000			
	Registrars (%)		Consultants (%)		Registrars (%)		Consultants (%)	
All	9 900	(100)	15 838	(100)	12 165	(100)	23 045	(100)
White	3 937	(40)	8 289	(52)	7 741	(64)	18 349	(80)
Black	380	(4)	240	(2)	565	(5)	755	(3)
Asian	880	(9)	679	(4)	2 782	(23)	2 141	(9)
Other	812	(8)	623	(4)	956	(8)	1 507	(7)
Unknown	3 890	(39)	6 007	(38)	121	(1)	293	(1)

(*Source*: Department of Health Statistics)

Focusing on consultants, where a similar high level of 'Unknowns' existed in 1991, the percentage of doctors from an ethnic minority background changes little in 2000. The number of consultants classifying themselves as 'White' has risen from 52% to 80%. The data suggest that much of the 'Unknown' group has been identified as 'White', and that consequently there has been little change in the overall makeup of the consultant group despite numerically higher numbers from ethnic minorities. Given the number of variables, other interpretations are possible for changes during these 10 years. However, because of the relative stability of the medical workforce and limited places to function outside the NHS system, interpretations can be made with a degree of confidence. The significant change in the registrar demographics, compared with little movement in those of the consultant, is partly answerable by the length of medical training. This leads to a time lag between the change in the registrar population and that of consultants.

Little data were available on the ethnic make-up of the primary care workforce and therefore a review of this is not possible. Turning to the gender profile, data are available about primary care (Table 9.2).

Table 9.2: Comparison of gender of GP registrars and GPs: 1990 and 2002

Gender	1990		2002	
	Registrars (%)	GPs (%)	Registrars (%)	GPs (%)
All	100	100	100	100
Female	48	25	62	37
Male	52	75	38	63

(*Source*: RCGP Information Sheet No. 1: Profile of UK General Practitioners – July 2003)

There has been a significant shift in the demographic make-up of both registrar and GP gender status. Female registrars have increased from 48% of the 1990 population to 62% in 2002, representing an additional 14% of the total registrar population. This significantly exceeds the percentage of woman studying medicine and dentistry in higher education, which stands at 55%.[12] Similarly, there has been a significant increase in the number of female GPs from 25% in 1990 to 37% in 2002, representing an additional 12% of the GP workforce. The higher number of female registrars suggests that the GP gender balance will move closer to a 50/50 balance sometime in the not too distant future.

Turning to the secondary care workforce, a similar significant increase in female registrars can be noted in conjunction with a significant increase in overall registrar numbers. The increase between 1991 and 2000 is from 26% to 37% of the registrar population (Table 9.3). Effectively, this is an increase of more than 40% in the numbers of female registrars over 10 years. Female consultants have increased from 16% to 22% of their work group over the same period. Again,

Table 9.3: Comparison of gender of registrars and consultants: 1991 and 2000

Gender	1991				2000			
	Registrars (%)		Consultants (%)		Registrars (%)		Consultants (%)	
All	9 900	(100)	15 838	(100)	12 165	(100)	23 045	(100)
Female	2 594	(26)	2 540	(16)	4 530	(37)	5 115	(22)
Male	7 306	(74)	13 298	(84)	7 635	(63)	17 930	(78)

(*Source*: Department of Health Statistics)

this is the context of a large increase in consultant numbers, which tends to mask the doubling of the female consultant population.

The purpose of this analysis is not to refute or support concerns of discrimination. Such findings would require far more detailed breakdowns of the figures viewed in the context of national developments and analysed for differences at speciality level and functional responsibilities. What these figures do show is a clear challenge for postgraduate education. The demographics of the trainers and the trainees are markedly different and undergoing considerable change at a time when social expectations are changing as well. Consequently, cultural and gender sensitivity in the delivery of postgraduate medical and dental education is essential to ensuring the full participation of all trainees and the development of a representative consultant and GP workforce.

Adverse impact or discrimination in medical education

Against this backdrop of significant changes in the gender and ethnic make-up of the medical workforce it is understandable that concerns about unfair discrimination arose. During the 1980s and 1990s a number of research articles and reports raised concern about the success rates of applicants from ethnic minorities to enter medical schools.[13] As well as at medical school level, an adverse impact was noted during the early part of the careers of women and junior doctors from ethnic minorities.[14] An 'adverse impact' occurs when a particular group performs notably below the norm for all students. It should be noted, however, that findings of unlawful racial and sexual discrimination do not automatically follow a finding of adverse impact, although objective justification for the difference will be necessary. So is there discrimination? What is the reality?

Research studies by Collier and Broke[15] and by McManus et al.[16] were among the earliest to highlight adverse impact on students from ethnic minority backgrounds in their applications for entry to medical school. More recently, research by McManus[17] highlighted that women are now more likely to gain a place at medical school but that ethnic minority candidates were still disadvantaged. McManus also produced evidence that the disadvantage to ethnic minorities is not uniform and varies based on ethnic category. In addition, adverse impact based on age and socio-economic background were also identified. The issue of age is particularly significant given impending legislation addressing age discrimination.

Although, as stated, adverse impact is not automatically an indicator of racial, sexual or other discrimination, there is a body of evidence supporting such concerns. A formal report by the CRE found discrimination in the appointment of NHS consultants and senior registrars.[18] A report by the King's Fund also raised concerns that more than 60% of doctors working in non-consultant career-grade posts are held by doctors from ethnic minorities. In addition, black and Asian doctors, especially those trained overseas, are more likely to end up working in unpopular specialities.[19]

Esmail and Everington[20] sent matched pairs of curriculum vitae, one with an English name and one an Asian name, in response to 23 advertisements for SHO positions. The applicants with English names were more likely to be shortlisted. Meanwhile, research by the Royal College of General Practitioners (RCGP) identified that women were under-represented in general practice teaching posts. In 1998 there were only four woman chairs of general practice in British university GP departments. Less than 5% of directors of GP education or postgraduate deans were women, and there were similar low figures for course organisers and GP tutors.[21] Furthermore, there are concerns that improvement in the numbers of women in medicine is not translating into equality of opportunity. Whereas 55% of students applying to British medical schools are female, it has been noted that only 6% of consultant surgeons are women.[22]

Some of these figures may have improved since they were published. There has been much work carried out by deaneries, by the GMC, the royal colleges, medical schools and the NHS generally to address concerns. This situation presents a challenge to postgraduate medical and dental education to ensure and to demonstrate that in the critical area of junior doctor training there is an education process which is free from unlawful discrimination. To do this the demographics of the trainees, trainers and networks managing postgraduate education need to be as representative as possible of diversity in the relevant populations.

Equalities in practice

In postgraduate medical and dental education, selection and assessment are two key areas where discrimination concerns are brought to the fore. This is unsurprising given the importance of these two processes in controlling entry and successful exit from the education system. Much of the early generic literature on fairness considered the issue of criterion validity, that is, do tests predict performance in the job. However, in the last 20 years there has been increased interest in how people perceive fairness, broadening the issue to consider social justice and individual perception. Performance is not only a function of skills and abilities, but is influenced by individual preferences, attitudes and expectations. Derous and De Witte[23] theorised that belief about the fairness of selection and assessment system will affect the test performance and even subsequent beliefs about self-efficacy, for example after recruitment. The basic concept is that, for example, applicants' perceptions influence their emotional reaction to the selection outcome that, in turn, influences cognitive processes, attitudes and behaviour.

The theory of organisational justice has been applied to the selection process and has identified the important role that process plays in individuals' judgement of fairness. The theory differentiates between *distributive* justice, the allocation of outcomes, and *procedural* justice, how these outcomes are reached.[24] Research has demonstrated that there are distinct but interlinked judgements on the receipt, or not, of a desired outcome and whether the process which resulted in the outcome was fair. It is possible for an individual to consider an outcome fair even though it is not personally positive.

Other research has considered assessment tests, where there has been a long-running concern about adverse effects on individuals from minority ethnic groups. Hough *et al.*[25] carried out a meta-analysis of adverse impact research. Whilst a full standard deviation difference was found with general intelligence tests, lower level cognitive abilities (such as verbal, quantitative and spatial awareness) can have lower levels of adverse impact. In addition, this impact was not the same for all minority ethnic groups.

Research in the UK by Dewberry in 2001[26] supports research findings in the USA of the lower performance of ethnic minority candidates. A selection process for trainee solicitors was used, in which some elements of the testing were marked blind. Analysis of selectors' decisions in both blind-marked and non-blind-marked tests found no evidence of discrimination. However, level of performance varied between ethnic minority groups, with older ethnic minority legal trainees more likely to have lower assessments than white legal trainees of the same age. This suggests that the prior experiences of the two groups differed. Correlates of higher assessments included good class of degree, going to 'Oxbridge' and not going to a new university. All these findings suggest that wider social and educational factors may affect the assessment of minority ethnic group candidates. Given these external factors, it is possible to see the argument for taking a wider social perspective of selection and assessment fairness.

Ultimately, not everyone will receive the outcome they want, and this is inevitable. What is important is that it is possible to explain why, and to demonstrate that the outcomes are discrimination-free. It is, however, equally important that the processes managed are seen to be fair. This requires an active engagement with all trainees, including good feedback and careers advice, fair and transparent procedures, policies that address and promote the principles of diversity, and research and review to support the selection and assessment processes.

Integrating diversity into the medical curriculum

It would be a mistake to consider equalities and diversity issues as an add-on to postgraduate medical and dental education. There is a clear need to mainstream these issues into teaching and learning. These are integral parts of the practice of medicine and the delivery of quality healthcare. Listed below are some areas where diversity issues have been highlighted in relation to healthcare and action taken or proposed. These are offered as brief examples of a complex issue.

Gender

The successful delivery of healthcare to a diverse population requires medical staff to be aware of the differing needs of individuals and groups. Men and women have specific healthcare needs that relate to their biological difference, for example contraception and childbirth for women. However, their needs are not simply biological but also arises from their social gender, which strongly influences living and working conditions. This is equally so for men whose pattern of access to healthcare is very different from that of women with a consequent negative effect on health.[27] Yet, the NHS has been criticised for not mainstreaming gender needs and ensuring that its workforce is properly trained.[28] This is a considerable educational challenge to the NHS, and has a potential impact on all users.

Age discrimination

Figures from the Department of Work and Pensions show that there are 18.6 million people aged 50 and over in the UK. About 10 million are over the state retirement age (60 for women, 65 for men), although not all are retired.[29] In its *National Service Framework for Older People*, published in 2001,[30] the Government recognised explicitly that the NHS was failing to meet the special needs of older people, who are a growing group and cross gender and ethnicity boundaries. These involve complex health needs, including physical, mental and social aspects. A study by the King's Fund[31] of senior managers based in hospitals, primary care groups, community trusts and social services departments found that age discrimination was poorly understood but generally recognised as occurring. Unsurprisingly, a key recommendation was for greater investment in the training and education of staff.

Multiprofessionalism

The role of the multiprofessional team is recognised to be a valuable factor in the provision of quality healthcare. This is recognised in *The NHS Plan*[5], in which new ways of working, professional demarcations and role development are addressed. Postgraduate medical and dental education has responded by promoting the benefits of multiprofessional teaching and learning to complement and support multiprofessional service delivery. This will continue to be an area attracting great interest and development.

Ethnicity

The 'Improving Health Among Ethnic Minority Populations'[32] initiative was developed in 1997. The programme was designed to assist the NHS to establish ways of meeting ethnic health needs within the mainstream agenda for addressing inequalities. The lessons from the projects are that if the health of minority ethnic groups is to be embedded in mainstream NHS service delivery it will have to be incorporated:

- in the infrastructure, as demonstrated by the patient profiling work
- across the whole system
- in partnership with other agencies
- in planning and specifying service requirements
- in developing and delivering appropriate treatment and health promotion.

This means working simultaneously at different levels within an organisation to address:

- individual awareness, competence and skills that need to be built and developed to give all staff the skills and confidence to address black and minority ethnic health issues
- organisational capacity and capability to deliver the expected gains in health for black and minority communities
- the need for a deeper understanding of the ways in which current health policy and practice interacts with race and ethnicity, that is, better knowledge of the issues to be addressed.

The educational and learning components of any plan to address equalities issues in service delivery are clear from the above examples. Deaneries have a crucial role in advising on, promoting and supporting initiatives to mainstream diversity issues into medical and dental curricula.

Final thoughts

The pace of change has accelerated dramatically. Changes in society and organisational change in the NHS generally and in postgraduate medical and dental education specifically have coalesced to present new challenges around equalities. Impending age discrimination legislation, Article 14, international recruitment and asylum-seeking doctors and dentists are just some examples. These challenges need to be grasped and managed in a clear and positive manner if medical education is to move forward in the UK in the 21st century.

References

1 McDougall M (1996) Equal opportunities versus managing diversity. Another challenge for public sector management? *International Journal of Public Sector Management.* **9**: 62–72.

2 Jehn KA, Northcraft GB and Neale M (1999) Why differences make a difference: a field study of diversity, conflict and performance in work groups. *Administrative Science Quarterly.* **44**: 741–63.

3 Anderson T and Metcalf H *(2003) Diversity: stacking up the evidence.* Chartered Institute of Personnel and Development, London.

4 General Medical Council (2001) *Good Medical Practice.* GMC, London.

5 Department of Health (2002) *The NHS Plan. A Plan for Investment. A Plan for Reform.* (CM 4818-I) DoH, London.

6 Department of Health (2001) *Shifting the Balance of Power. Securing Delivery.* DoH, London.

7 Department of Health (2002) *Promoting Equality and Diversity in the NHS: a guide for board members.* Crown Copyright. (www.doh.gov.uk/publicationsandstatistics)

8 Commission for Racial Equality (2002) *Framework for a Race Equality Policy – For Higher Education.* CRE, London. (www.cre.gov.uk)

9 Equal Opportunities Commission (1998) *Gender and Differential Achievement in Education and Training: a research review.* Equal Opportunities Commission, Manchester. (www.eoc.org.uk)

10 Office of National Statistics (1997) *Labour Force Survey, Spring 1997.* ONS, London.

11 Higher Education Statistics Agency (1995) *Ethnicity in Higher Education.* HESA, Cheltenham. (www.hesa.ac.uk)

12 Higher Education Statistics Agency (2002) *All HE Students by Subject of Study, Domicile and Gender 2001/02.* HESA, Cheltenham. (www.hesa.ac.uk)

13 Mckenzie KJ (1995) Racial discrimination in medicine (Editorial). *BMJ.* **310**: 478–9.

14 McKeigue PM, Richards JDM and Richards P (1990) Effects of discrimination by sex and race on early careers of British medical graduates during 1981–7. *BMJ.* **301**: 961–4.

15 Collier J and Broke A (1986) Racial and sexual discrimination in the selection of students for London medical schools. *Medical Education.* **20**: 86–90.

16 McManus IC, Richards P and Maitlis SL (1989) Prospective study of the disadvantage of people from ethnic minority groups applying to medical schools in the United Kingdom. *BMJ.* **298**: 723–6.

17 McManus IC (1998) Factors affecting likelihood of applicants being offered a place in medical schools in the United Kingdom in 1996 and 1997; retrospective study. *BMJ.* **317**: 1111–7.

18 Commission for Racial Equality (1996) *Appointing NHS Consultants and Senior Registrars: report of a formal investigation.* CRE, London.

19 Coker N (2001) *Racism in Medicine: an agenda for change.* King's Fund, London.

20 Esmail A and Everington S (1993) Racial discrimination against doctors from ethnic minorities. *BMJ.* **310**: 496–500.

21 Royal College of General Practitioners (1998) *The RCGP Information Sheet; Women General Practitioners.* RCGP, London.

22 McDonald R (2002) Discrimination in medicine. *BMJ.* **324**: 1112.

23 Derous E and De Witte K (2001) Looking at selection from a social process perspective: towards a social process model on personnel selection. *European Journal of Work and Organizational Psychology.* **10**: 319–42.

24 Gilliland SW (1993) The perceived fairness of selection systems: an organisational justice perspective. *Academy of Management Review.* **18**: 694–734.

25 Hough LM., Oswald FL and Ployhart RE (2001) Determinants, detection and amelioration of adverse impact in personnel selection procedures: issues, evidence and lessons learned. *International Journal of Selection and Assessment.* **9**: 152–94.

26 Dewberry C (2001) Performance disparities between whites and ethnic minorities: real differences or assessment bias? *Journal of Occupational and Organizational Psychology.* **74**: 659–73.

27 Banks I (2001) No man's land: men, illness, and the NHS. *BMJ.* **323**: 1058–60.

28 Doyal L, Payne S and Cameron A (2003) *Promoting Gender Equality in Health.* School for Policy Studies, University of Bristol; Equal Opportunities Commission, London. (www.eoc.org.uk)

29 Department of Work and Pensions (2001) *Labour Force Survey Autumn 2001.* Department of Work and Pensions, London.

30 Department of Health (2001) *National Service Framework for Older People.* LAC (2001)12. Crown Copyright. Department of Health, London.

31 Roberts E, Robinson J and Seymour L (2002) *Old Habits Die Hard: tackling age and discrimination in health and social care.* King's Fund, London.

32 Department of Health (1997) *Improving Health Among Ethnic Minority Populations.* Crown Copyright. DoH, London. (www.doh.gov.uk)

CHAPTER 10

E-learning

Shelley Heard

Introduction

Since the Open University (OU) first set the tone in the UK for distance learning in the 1960s, the potential to use technology to support learning has become widely used. In recent years there has been a rapid expansion in the use of e-learning in almost every aspect of teaching and education. The OU now reports that some 180 000 students interact with its learning programmes every week.[1]

Medicine has been quick to identify opportunities to use the advantages afforded by e-learning to give improved access and to share a wide range of learning opportunities. Virtual learning environments are becoming commonplace at both undergraduate and postgraduate level. The previous commitment of the Department of Health to develop the NHS University (NHSU)[2] to support learning for NHS staff indicates that there will be significant investment to support e-learning opportunities.

What is e-learning?

Learning through the opportunities afforded by the internet, CD-ROMs and other electronic means enables a new approach to developing and delivering learning. It is not restricted to time or to place; learners can have increased flexibility to learn where and when they wish, to repeat and review aspects of the learning material and to focus on particular areas of interest. The NHSU identified the benefits of e-learning for individuals and for organisations as follows.

- For individuals: e-learning can empower individuals to learn, achieve and progress by giving them easy access to learning opportunities and support.
- For managers: e-learning can help managers to achieve their targets by developing teams and individuals with the right knowledge and skills.
- For health professionals: e-learning enables collaboration and communication by creating online communities.

- For organisations: e-learning can help organisations to work with each other to develop their staff and manage knowledge.
- For carers: e-learning offers carers an opportunity to learn from home and to communicate with other carers.
- For patients: e-learning can help individual and communities to become partners in learning and raise standards of care.

E-learning and learning styles?

Not all learning, and not all learners, are suitable for e-learning. A report, commissioned by the NHS Information Authority, from the University of Salford[3] makes the important point that e-learning may not necessarily be the optimal way to meet a training need. It recommends that a key step in thinking about creating an e-learning opportunity is to ensure that an appropriate learning or training needs analysis is undertaken. This is critical in order to evaluate whether the development of an e-learning approach to a particular learning problem is the most appropriate one to take.[4]

One of the most frequently identified models of learning used to describe how we learn is Kolb's experiential learning.[5] This well-known learning cycle describes four elements to learning, as follows.

- *Experiencing*, in which the task assigned is carried out either by the organisation or the individual – what Kolb describes as 'immersing yourself in the task'.
- *Reflection*, requires stepping back from the task being undertaken and thinking about what is being done, verbalising, and if possible, discussing what is going on. It requires thinking and putting into context the learning that is being undertaken.
- *Conceptualisation*, about interpreting events and trying to understand the relationships between them.
- *Planning*, involves the learner in considering what action should be taken in order to use the learning and move forward.

Considering learning in this way enables learners, including organisations, to learn from experience and to develop as a result. Honey and Mumford[6] have used this model to identify four learning preferences, as follows.

- *Activists* are learners who 'like to have a go and see what happens'. They like to share different experiences and to learn with others, but learn less well through lectures, being asked to merely take in data or by working on their own.
- *Reflectors* prefer to gather information and think about things. They learn by observation and like to review and consider what has happened but learn less well if they do not have time to prepare or are pushed to meet deadlines.

- *Theorists* like to take information and draw conclusions from it in a logical and clear way. They learn by questioning and thinking through complex problems, but do not learn well if learning is unstructured or if they do not understand the underlying principles. They also find it difficult to learn with people who do not learn in a similar way.
- *Pragmatists* like to use already tried-and-tested strategies which can deal with the problem being considered. They do well in learning situations where they can receive feedback and also learn well from practising models that have been shown to be successful. They do less well if the learning is only theory and if there are no immediate benefits achieved.

So, it is important for people who develop e-learning materials to be aware that not all of it will necessarily be accessible to all learners, and equally, for learners to be cognisant of what is likely to be appropriate for them. Content also needs to be developed for learners who learn visually, where graphics and animation support their learning, for those who learn best through listening (auditory learners) and who need to interact with others, possibly through chatrooms, case studies and interacting, or for kinaesthetic learners, who need 'movement' with lots of functionality and online exercises.[7]

What are the advantages of e-learning?

Much has been written about e-learning. It has been taken up by business and corporations in order to enhance company performance through developing and supporting the workforce. Cross, one of the leading e-learning gurus in the USA, has described it thus:

> e-learning is learning on internet time, the convergence of learning and networks and the New Economy. e-learning is a vision of what corporate training can become ... e-learning is to traditional training as e-business is to business as usual. Both use the net to augment traditional means ... [in the context of corporate learning] effective e-learning dramatically cuts the time it takes for people to become and remain competent in their jobs.[8]

E-learning focuses on the need of the learner rather than the organisation or institution. It improves access both geographically and in terms of real-time availability. Learners are able to explore a range of learning approaches and pace their own learning. There is the ability for learners to learn with their peer group through chat rooms, collaborative learning projects and discussion groups. Educational facilitators who are well trained and available can support learners in an online environment. Educational support activities, such as information on how to access online material, how the virtual learning environment works, registration and assessment of progress, are all part of the package.

What does all this mean for the NHS?

The NHS is the biggest employer in the UK, with some 1.5 million employees. Training and supporting learning in a range of complex environments for individuals with a huge divergence of learning needs, involving specific knowledge, skills and attitudinal aspects of learning is extremely challenging. Demonstrating the impact of such learning on the delivery of patient care – the 'end-product' of NHS business – is even more so. The commitment of the NHS to supporting lifelong learning was made clear in the publication of *Working Together, Learning Together: a framework for lifelong learning in the NHS*,[9] published by the Department of Health in 2001. In the Foreword to the document the Secretary of State, Alan Milburn, made it clear that:

> Learning and development are key to delivering the Government's vision of patient-centred care in the NHS. Lifelong learning is about growth and opportunity, about making sure that our staff, the teams and organisations they relate to, and work in, can acquire new knowledge and skills, both to realise their potential and to help shape and change things for the better. Lifelong learning is inextricably linked with the wider agenda for building, rewarding and supporting the NHS workforce for the future.

Lifelong learning involves a commitment from NHS employers to ensure that learning opportunities are made available to all staff to support their own development within the context of the work that they do. E-learning provides the potential to support this ambitious aim. The NHSU is an important part of that strategy. Its plan to develop a virtual learning campus, which will enable users to access a range of e-learning materials both at work and at home, should significantly enhance the possibilities of lifelong learning but also affords the opportunity to enhance service and patient care.

The NHSU successor body, the new NHS Institute for Learning, Skills and Innovation (Nilsi) (*see* Chapter 2), will continue to emphasise the importance of lifelong learning and e-learning in the NHS.

E-learning in the NHS

There are a number of key areas where e-learning is already making an impact in the NHS.

Professional staff

For clinicians there are numerous speciality-specific sites that support learners in developing their knowledge and skills. These are variable in their source and in their scope; some are free but many require a registration and a fee. It is important that care is taken to know the source and the reliability of the content, but, in the UK, sites from the Royal Colleges offer not only information about the services and support offered by the Colleges, but often learning material as well. Professional development opportunities are offered through more generic sites, which are now producing a wide range of short duration learning 'sound-bites'.[10,11] E-learning diagnostic support systems are also available, and these help clinicians in the clinical environment to review patients in real time.[12] Online learning opportunities are also available to support generic skills training for healthcare professionals.[13]

Patients

For patients as well there are numerous sites available to provide information about a range of healthcare issues. This is of particular benefit to patients and carers with long-term chronic clinical conditions, such as diabetes[14] and Parkinson's disease,[15] although information on virtually any condition can be found on the Internet. Patients increasingly bring their growing knowledge to the attention of their clinicians, where this sort of e-learning supports the clinical consultation process and can, as well, enhance the development of the patient–clinician partnership.

Organisations

The potential for e-learning to enhance appropriate, relevant and timely learning is a major attraction for employers. The need for courses and facilitated learning is not replaced by e-learning opportunities, but can be supported and enhanced by the availability of electronic learning materials. Most organisations seek an approach using 'blended' or mixed learning, which exploits e-learning resources, for both learning materials and when using online teacher support – along with a variety of facilitated face-to-face learning approaches. The NHSU has developed courses, for example, an induction programme called 'Working for the NHS', which has elements of e-learning as well as taught components, but its 'Advanced Communication in Cancer Care' course does not involve any e-learning.

Organisations can also use e-learning to support service initiatives and change. Two good examples of this are the potential to use e-learning programmes to support activities such as the 'Hospital at Night'[16] initiative, which seeks to find new and better ways of supporting patient care outside of the working day, and the 'Changing Workforce' programme[17] which explores different ways of delivering healthcare services by identifying new roles and areas of work. In turn, not only can managers and organisations share information about such key changes electronically, but specific learning programmes can be also be delivered electronically to support them[18] and to support clinical educators within the service.[19]

Summary

The development and use of e-learning materials is clearly not an end in itself. E-learning provides educational tools that can be used to improve access to educational material and learning opportunities. Its ongoing technical development and an improved understanding of the way in which it can be integrated with facilitated, face-to-face learning and educator support are essential future developments.

References

1 www.open.ac.uk

2 www.nhsu.org

3 NHS Information Authority (2003) *Guidelines to Inform the Development of e-learning in the NHS*. Research study by the University of Salford. NHS Information Authority, London.

4 Broadbent B (2003) *Selecting Training to Deliver in an E-learning Mode*. 2003 (Accessed 2004: www.e-learninghub.com/articles/selecting_training.html)

5 Kolb DA (1984) *Experiential Learning: experience as the source of learning and development.* Prentice Hall, New Jersey.

6 Campaign for Learning: what kind of learner are you? From Honey P and Mumford A (1982) *The Learning Questionnaire.* (Accessed 2004: www.campaign-for-learning.org.uk/aboutyour learning/whatlearning.htm)

7 Summers L (year) *Multiple Learning Styles in Web-based Courses.* (Accessed 2004: www.webct.com/service/viewcontentframe?contentID=2334144)

8 Cross J (2002) *The e Learning FAQ.* (Accessed 2004: www.internettime.com/Learning/faq.htm)

9 Department of Health (2001) *Working Together, Learning Together: a framework for lifelong learning in the NHS*. DoH, London. (www.publications.doh.gov.uk/lifelonglearning/index.htm)

10 www.bmjlearning.com

11 www.doctors.net.uk

12 www.isabel.org.uk

13 www.healthcareskills.nhs.uk

14 www.diabetes.org/home.jsp

15 www.parkinsons.org.uk

16 www.modern.nhs.uk/hospitalatnight/

17 www.modernnhs.nhs.uk/scripts/default.asp?site_id=65

18 Conference of Postgraduate Medical Deans (2002) *Report of the Conference of Postgraduate Medical Deans ad hoc Working Group on the Educational Implications of the European Working Time Directive.* (www.copmed.org.uk/Publications/liberatinglearning/index.html (document)) (www.liberatinglearning.nhs.uk (web-based programme)).

19 www.clinicalteaching.nhs.uk

CHAPTER 11

Higher professional education for new GPs

Neil Jackson and Tareq Abouharb

Introduction

The concept of higher professional education (HPE) for newly qualified general practitioners (GPs) has been established for a number of years. HPE may be considered as the provision of additional support to help newly qualified GPs in their transition from GP Registrar to established independent practice as a GP. It is now generally accepted that this provision should be given for at least a two-year period after completion of basic vocational training.

The role of HPE is multifaceted. By its very nature it aims to give formative focus to the new GP's ongoing development of reflective practice. In addition to providing some of the financial support and time out for individuals to pursue their personal development agenda, it gives a forum for peer support and interaction. The hope is that this combination will contribute to the development of settled GPs, who are more likely to remain within their locality, take up more permanent posts and thus enhance recruitment and retention.

The postgraduate training of doctors in the UK is undergoing a major review, as part of the 'Modernising Medical Careers' (MMC) agenda. The development of a specialist training 'run–through' grade with an integral role for HPE in its latter stages for the evolving GP is an exciting prospect. With this in mind, this chapter aims to describe the strategic and operational challenges to the development of HPE thus far.

Historical background

The Royal College of General Practitioners (RCGP)[1] recommended in 1965 that GP vocational training should take place over a four-year period, thus emphasising the need for an appropriate length of training with adequate supervision and support to prepare young doctors for the realities of their future working lives in general practice.

Despite this, the NHS general practice vocational training regulations (which were established in 1979) specified that three years' full-time employment (or its part-time equivalent) were required to satisfy the regulations for prescribed experience. The three years would be made up of one year as a trainee general practitioner (GP registrar, GPR) and the remainder in hospital posts in fields which were considered appropriate for general practice training.

By the early 1990s it had become apparent that GPs were expected to fulfil an expanding role in the NHS. They needed to be adequately equipped for this new kind of job and it was realised that the basic three-year programme of GP vocational training could not be sufficient for the modern day GP. If the three-year envelope for GP training was to remain intact, there was then a need to establish a system of post-vocational training support in the form of an agreed framework for HPE.

The evidence base for higher professional education

In 1998, the Committee of General Practice Education Directors (COGPED) published its report on HPE.[2] The prevailing view, expressed in this report, was that many recently vocationally trained GP registrars would benefit from an additional one or two years of supervision and support in a suitable learning environment. This would increase their preparedness and fitness for their role through a number of approaches, for example:

- enhancing the development of research and teaching skills
- undertaking a masters degree course or similar higher qualification
- developing additional clinical skills
- enhancing information technology and management skills
- generally heightening awareness of the GP's role in the wider primary care context, including the complexities of the GPs enhanced role in providing and commissioning care for patients.

The important issue identified in the report was the provision of ongoing educational support at the start of a new GP's career to enhance both competence and confidence. Also, the report noted that although progress was being made in the provision of HPE for new GPs, with a variety of educational initiatives in different parts of the UK, there was a lack of a proper financial framework for making educational support available. This lack was impeding progress and further development.

The report also highlighted various aspects of what was thought to be the appropriate educational context of HPE. These included:

- learner-centredness

- personal learning plans
- the provision of mentoring
- peer group support
- Multiprofessional or multidisciplinary working.

The final report of the London Initiative Zone Educational Incentive scheme was also published in 1998.[3] This three-year programme of educational initiatives for general practice from 1995 to 1998 was set within a framework of the four 'Rs' – recruitment, retention, refreshment and reflection. The scheme itself offered many varied training opportunities. One of these, the London Academic Training Scheme (LATS),[4] is an excellent example of an HPE initiative. It offers an additional period of 12 months' academic training, together with support through a facilitated group for GP registrars following completion of the basic GP vocational training programme.

Also in 1998, an influential report was published by the Joint Centre for Education in Medicine.[5] This highlighted the problems with the transition from GP registrar to GP principal and an associated sudden reduction in educational supervision and support after completion of vocational training. The report illustrated the reluctance of newly qualified GPs to enter a principal post. It suggested that this cohort of doctors had further training needs. It recognised that there was a largely unstructured approach to facilitating their further training and development, without properly organised educational supervision and support.

Was this a problem primarily stemming from the length and educational content of the GP vocational training programme, which was not sufficient preparation for the new principal? If the vocational training programme was to be extended, what of the content and process of learning? Should it be more of the same or something entirely different? On the other hand, could it be that the basic vocational training programme was sufficient to enable most GP registrars to emerge at the end of the training period as competent GPs, in terms of basic knowledge and most clinical skills, but not 'fit for purpose'? Was a different emphasis, with supervision and support, required? This might be provided by a programme, the purpose of which was to enable newly qualified GPs to become 'fit for the purpose' of working in the primary care system of the NHS?

Health professionals become 'fit for purpose' when they are properly confident and competent to carry out what is regarded as appropriate healthcare provision in the modern setting. For a GP this means:

- having appropriate book knowledge and clinical skills
- knowing how to exercise this knowledge and skill
- knowing how to relate to patients
- knowing how to work in a team
- knowing how to provide services for groups of patients

- knowing how to maintain quality of practice
- knowing how to lay the foundations for lifelong learning.

Fitness for purpose is a concept that applies equally to individual healthcare professionals (in this case new GPs) and to the healthcare system in which they work. Both the workers and the organisation must be able to deliver a quality service for patients. The NHS itself must be fit for the purpose of helping the development of its workforce. In part it must do this by providing appropriate opportunities for professional development.

As our new generation of young GPs emerge from their vocational training, it is clear that not being 'fit for purpose' is a real problem. Their undergraduate curriculum may not have addressed the factual and life adaptation skills needed to deal with today's healthcare setting and pace of change. Yes, this deficit is being addressed by modernising the medical undergraduate curriculum. But, for today's young GPs, the new funding arrangements for protected time for learning at last give us a real opportunity to think about ways of helping post-vocationally trained GPs further develop themselves, so that fitness for purpose is achieved.

How can we, who are responsible for managing and facilitating these new opportunities for young GPs, best go about our task? We could, at one extreme, look to empower the new GP to explore how best to optimise self-directed learning. We could provide a model that is both more thoughtful and more academic (by academic we mean 'more enquiring, more evidence-based'). We might need to be responsible for the supervision of such reflective learning. Special emphasis would need to be devoted to the resolution of the immediate problems of young doctors, which are usually work-based. Such problems often stem from the real and live difficulties of working with patients. At the other end of the scale, we could offer a purely 'service provision model'. This would be an information-giving and training-based model. We could impart information to new GPs about patients' needs without addressing learners' developmental needs.

Our view is that this latter model would fall short in the long term, with its lack of reflective focus. The model of education, which this chapter will go on to describe, should look to balance the academic and service provision components. It will equip new GPs to move to a reflective self-directed learning method and provide the opportunity to gain and consolidate clinical knowledge and skill of value to the care of their patients.

The strategic importance of higher professional education

In strategic terms, HPE is of importance for both the recruitment and retention of competent GPs in the new NHS. A framework for HPE provision must be designed to withstand at least three clear challenges:

- meeting and supporting the educational needs of new GPs (the transition to independent practice)
- assisting new GPs in becoming fit for the purpose of working in the NHS
- enhancing the retention of new GPs in the GP workforce.

New Government funding for HPE came on stream on 1 October 2001, to be managed by directors of postgraduate general practice education (DsPGPE), and deaneries are now developing their support systems to reach the target group of new GPs. This has required an expansion of the deanery educational network by the appointment of programme directors to support HPE programmes and their participants under the leadership of a lead Associate Director of Postgraduate General Practice Education (ADPGPE).

Providing a strategic framework to improve locality recruitment and retention requires that policy takes account of the changing expectations and hopes of those completing vocational training. The evidence that new GPs look for flexible work patterns and initially prefer to engage in roles not requiring geographical or financial commitment is important in planning any supportive provision. A raft of measures offering new ways of working, such as the Flexible Career Scheme (FCS) and new ways of addressing learning needs, such as HPE, have begun to make the reality of modern general practice more approachable for new GPs. Ensuring the 'portability' of HPE support across deanery boundaries adds to its empowering effect. In making individual new GPs feel better supported and facilitating their personal and professional development, there are now encouraging signs that retention rates in areas with previously high 'net – exporter' profile, deploying these strategies are reducing egression and holding onto their precious New GP commodity for longer.

Operational developments in higher professional education

From the historical perspective already discussed in this chapter it can be seen how common themes in HPE, emerging from previous studies, could go on to shape the practicalities of a programme. The structure, content and process of such a programme – what will happen, who will do it, how it will be done and what its aim must be – form the basis of the operational development of HPE.

HPE structure

The structure of a programme for HPE is determined by previous experience[2] and the following key factors:

- national policy and the COGPED framework setting the standard

- funding limitations and the number of GPs that may be eligible to enter the scheme
- the educational needs of the GPs
- what the patients and primary care teams will tolerate in terms of reduction in service provision levels while educational needs are addressed for GPs
- geographical considerations, and sensitivities to locality service needs
- commitment to information technology (IT).

One of the first tasks is to identify new GPs and establish a database that can then support HPE delivery. This presents a number of practical problems because of concurrent changes within the NHS, in organisations managing the necessary data:

- the devolvement of health authority functions to primary care trusts (PCTs)
- the evolution of strategic health authorities (SHAs)
- the establishment of supplementary lists to identify non-principal GPs (some of whom will also be new GPs).

At a time of rapidly expanding personal computing access to the internet, the way in which deaneries support individuals needs to reflect modern IT practice. The convenience and speed IT offers individuals in such a setting may be crucial to the perception of being attuned to learners' needs. This may challenge the resources of educational bodies to have IT strategy match user expectations.

The HPE team

The HPE team facilitates delivery of HPE to new GPs, and locality programme development and delivery is the responsibility of programme directors. They are appointed and managed by the deanery. Their personal qualities, aptitudes and skills are vital for the success of their mission. Programme directors need to be good communicators and facilitators, have educational and clinical experience in primary care and an ability to network. They need to make a connection between vocational training schemes and continuing professional development (the arrangements for lifelong learning for established professionals), to ensure the supportive continuum highlighted earlier. They will also need support to discharge their task as well as time to interact with fellow educators with responsibility in this field. This will give them feedback and stimulate reflection on shared experience. Such a process should both help to generate best practice and inform strategic planning at deanery level. The HPE team works closely with others in the deanery through a 'GP Educator Development Group', which plan team development events. This enhances shared learning with other colleagues in the deanery educational network, and broadens the flavour of the experience within which new skills and knowledge are acquired.

HPE content

When new GPs assess their educational needs, it is interesting to see how consistent are the range of subjects raised.[5,6] This reflects the difficulties new GPs face in transition from the closely supported registrar post to fully fledged independent practice, with potential deficits in knowledge, clinical, management and coping skills. It must also be ensured that new GPs deal with issues of health strategy such as national service frameworks and their implementation within a new general medical services (GMS) contract. New GPs will also seek to develop areas of individual strength that may contribute to evolving a longer-term locality role, such as a GP with specialist interest (GPwSI). A working compilation of these into a proposed core curriculum for HPE can be seen in Appendix I.

Process of HPE delivery

The key to HPE delivery will be each individual's personal development plan (PDP), potentially linked with practice and wider needs and planning.[7] A learning needs assessment[8] forms the basis of planning for an individual's HPE activity and the advent of GP registrar appraisal gives new GPs an opportunity to review the outcomes of this process with their HPE Programme Director. The PDP needs to be responsive to the changing and newly identified needs, at a time of significant challenge and potential vulnerability. Helping new GPs to reflect on and prioritise their plans will, therefore, be an early component of the new GP–Programme Director interaction. Individuals will have unique needs and, for the process to be truly effective, it must be flexible enough to facilitate each individual's educational journey.

Modes of delivery

Although a range of educational vehicles has been suggested as a way of optimising HPE delivery,[5] an over-riding issue is to encourage new GPs to move on from the closely supervised model of vocational training scheme day release to a reflective, self-directed lifelong learning model.

Funding streams, as laid out in the COGPED framework of the national policy, have ensured a maximal 20 days of protected educational time for new GPs undertaking HPE, through service provision support for practices to seek locum cover. Funding to cover educational expenses is also set out. The national framework, although most welcome, proved to be somewhat limiting to HPE delivery by virtue of the realities of locum costs and educational expenses. The challenge here is how best to utilise these funds to:

- fully devolve ownership to individuals to direct as they choose

- target funds at specific activities, for example supporting self-directed learning groups
- develop some compromise, which would be overseen in partnership by new GPs and their programme directors.

The evolution of an individual learning account (ILA) format pilot, to facilitate the use of the funding so that it can better reflect the individual learning arrangements needed for PDPs is proving very helpful. Planned evaluation of the ILA pilot will help to clarify future strategy.

However these funds are used and whether new GPs learn within supportive groups, in supervised placements or on their own, the new GP's PDP will act as the key planning and evaluation document for the following year's educational activity. Each GP's PDP should be built on an awareness or assessment of his or her learning needs. The Programme Director will need to make personal contact with new GPs and start the process of facilitating this process.

This model has at its heart a dynamic learner-centred relationship between the programme director and the new GP. The relative numbers of new GP learners and programme directors is such that it will be difficult to have an exclusive one-to-one relationship here, although to some degree the relationship has to be facilitative and supervisory. Perhaps the elements of facilitation and supervision will occur most completely through peer groups. This solution does indeed build on others' experience in the post-vocational training scheme support setting. In the study by Bregazzi *et al.*, a one-to-one mentoring model for new GPs in their work setting proved problematic at times, whereas peer support and learning groups were more valued by the participating GPs. In summary, therefore, the proposal for HPE is based on the following.

- Educational supervision by a programme director of individual plans – this may not be done on a one-to-one basis and may need to be delegated.
- An emphasis on the peer- and self-directed learning group as a most appropriate way to facilitate the learning and development process.

As with colleagues in other deaneries planning delivery of HPE, we need to understand how to develop the role of these groups and of individual new GPs within them.[10] The programme director will need to be facilitative in order to stimulate debate and negotiation in the group so that it can arrive at the most supportive arrangement.

With the bones of the model now outlined, it may be valuable to clarify the learning process and the supportive structure. New GPs are under a professional imperative to ensure that they keep up to date with skills and knowledge and become fit for purpose. The programme director provides educational supervision and facilitation. They may pass this duty on to a third party (for example, a consultant where the young doctor is sitting in during clinics). Equally, that third party may be a peer-learning group. So, supervision and support may well be shared with this third party in the setting of an individual new GP's secondment or with a learning group that incorporates peer support and supervision. This flexibility thus allows the programme director to both ensure that learners' needs are addressed and that the learning process takes place in the most appropriate setting.

Programme directors need many skills because they are the gate-keepers of the scheme. They will need to maintain the quality and credibility of the educational activity, whilst keeping the option of the mode of delivery firmly in the hands of the learner.

Although new GPs may have learning needs not presently addressed in CPD provision, encouraging them to take up existing CPD opportunities that are relevant may serve to reduce the sense of isolation otherwise engendered in learning only as part of an HPE group. CPD will put them in touch with experienced colleagues whose knowledge base would offer a valuable resource, and potential contacts for future support network.

HPE and modern general practice

Over the past 20 years there has been a dramatic shift in both the expectations of doctors and their patients of how primary care delivery and its associated educational support should function. This generation of new GPs has grown up and entered the profession since the change in GP contractual regulations in 1990, and many are now joining just in time to face the uncharted challenges of the new GMS contract. They often accept that change must occur, but are less accepting of how work in general might affect the quality of their personal and family lives. More females are now choosing a career in primary care, and a greater proportion of them are choosing to work part-time.[11]

This change in culture may have been accelerated by a combination of increasing stressors and greater choice. The stressors take the form of increasing litigation, reduction in perceived kudos and ever-increasing workload. The choice being that the MB BS qualification may now open doors to other careers with equal, if not better, rates of pay, which potentially generate less angst.

Thus, HPE is entering the fray at a critical time for recruitment and retention. It may offer a shield to protect new GPs from some of the stressors while they develop survival skills. It may also act to bolster new GPs' self-worth as they acquire skills that are relevant to their future practice or to their work within the primary care team. HPE must go some way to addressing these issues. The majority of individuals opt for a career in general practice once they have qualified as a doctor.[12] It is therefore important that the positive view they take of this option is maintained through the difficult period of transition after the vocational training scheme.

Support and supervision for the learning and development of new GPs is important as it recognises the value of the individual within the NHS. It should help to move GPs towards becoming self-directed learners and establish a reflective approach to personal development. To develop individuals in this way has been the secret of many a successful organisation.

It is in the challenge of delivering HPE that one begins to see the effects of the cultural shift in attitudes to the role and lifestyle of modern day GPs. Resolving the tension between one's personal life and the demands of work is one part of the formula, but we must ensure that there are appropriate opportunities for self-development and for becoming 'fit for purpose' so that GPs remain committed and enthusiastic about their chosen work.

As primary care evolves and postgraduate education looks to frameworks such as MMC to respond better to the needs of the NHS and the doctors within it, the need to encourage and support clinicians and feed this experience back into the evolving strategy of the profession has never been greater. Our professional and accreditation bodies will need to support, lead and challenge us to move the agenda forwards.

Appendix I: Proposed core curriculum for HPE

Performance

- Appraisal and personal development planning
- Preparing for revalidation
- Practice professional development plans
- Clinical governance/HImP/NSF.

Skills

- IT or presentation skills
- Consultation skills/Communication skills/Creative problem-solving
- Negotiation skills and assertiveness training/Time and stress management
- Audit and research
- Report writing
- Secondary care provision in primary care
- Information gathering/Critical reading skills
- Practising evidence-based medicine
- Medicine and the law:
  - Partnership agreements/Joining a practice
  - Medico-legal dilemmas
  - Ethical dilemmas
  - Contractual agreements in the modern NHS (GMS/PMS, etc.)
- Practice management and finance:

- – Practice management/Recruitment and Employment Law
- – Personal finance
- – Practice finance/accounts and Claims
- Self-directed personal development/Supervision/Reflective learning
  - – Career planning
  - – Mentoring
  - – Optimising self-directed learning/Self-directed learning groups
  - – Higher degrees/Support for education

References

1 Royal College of General Practitioners (1965) *Report of a Working Party of Special Vocational Training for General Practice.* RCGP, London.

2 Jackson N and Reiss M (1998) *Higher Professional Education for General Practice: report on current work in the UK based on completed questionnaires from directors of postgraduate general practice.* COGPED, London.

3 NHS Executive (1998) *London Initiative Zone Educational Incentive (LIZEI) Scheme Final Report (Recruitment, Retention refreshment, Refreshment and Reflection).* NHS Executive, London.

4 Freeman G (1997) LATS Second Annual Report 1996–1997. Imperial College School of Medicine, London.

5 Joint Centre for Education in Medicine *An Evaluation of Educational Needs and Provision for Doctors within Three Years of Completion of Vocational Training for General Practice.* JCEM, London.

6 Baron R, Mckinlay D, Martin J, *et al.* (2001) Higher professional education for GPs in the north west of England – feedback from the first three years. *Education for Primary Care.* **12**: 421–9.

7 Department of Health (1998) *A First Class Service: quality in the new NHS.* HMSO, London.

8 Grant J (2002) Learning needs assessment: assessing the need. *BMJ.* **324**:156–9.

9 Bregazzi R, Harrison J and Van Zwanenberg T (2000) Mentoring new GPs: experience from GP Career Start in County Durham. *Education for General Practice.* **11**: 58–64.

10 Rughani A, Tomson M, McFarlane A *et al.* (2002) Continuous professional development – help for new GPs. *Update.* **May**: 742–5.

11 Royal College of General Practitioners (1997) *The Primary Care Workforce. A Descriptive Analysis.* RCGP, London.

12 Bowler I and Jackson N (2002) Experiences and career intentions of general practice registrars in Thames deaneries. *BMJ.* **324**: 464–5.

CHAPTER 12

Attracting doctors to the NHS

Penny Trafford, Yong-Lock Ong and Ian Hastie

Introduction

The majority of doctors trained in the UK will work in the National Health Service (NHS); however, at present there is a shortage. Many doctors want to come to this country to work from abroad and we have to have processes in place to enable them to do this. At the same time we have to find ways of encouraging doctors already here to either stay in the NHS or return to it.

Regulations and training

There are regulations determining whether doctors from countries outside the UK are allowed to work in the UK and undergo postgraduate training. The following are the definitions of non-UK doctors used in this chapter.

Overseas doctors

Doctors who do not have a right to indefinite residence in the UK. This includes doctors who hold a primary medical qualification from a UK university, but do not have the right of indefinite residence in the UK

Overseas-qualified doctors

Doctors who have taken their primary medical qualification outside the European Economic Association (EEA).

Refugee doctors

Doctors who have taken their primary medical qualification outside the EEA and also have refugee status, indefinite leave to remain or humanitarian status.

EEA doctors

Doctors whose primary medical qualification or postgraduate qualification is from an EEA country.

General Medical Council

All doctors coming from abroad to work in the NHS must confirm with the General Medical Council (GMC) that they are eligible for registration.

Overseas doctors who wish to apply for registration with the GMC must demonstrate that they have the necessary knowledge of English by passing the International English Language Testing System (IELTS) examation,[1] which is administered by the British Council. The GMC will also provide advice on whether the overseas doctor needs to pass the test run by the Professional and Linguistics Assessment Board (PLAB). This test is a broad-based examination, in two parts, designed to ensure that overseas doctors are competent to practise in the UK at the level of a first-year senior house officer (SHO) in any of the main branches of medicine and surgery. There are a small number of overseas trainees who are supported by colleges for PLAB exemption within a named speciality. These doctors seem to have greater difficulty obtaining SHO jobs in open competition in highly competitive specialities and, for many overseas doctors, it is preferable to pass the PLAB examination, which allows them to apply for jobs in all specialities.

The GMC is in the process of reviewing the rules around registration. However, as this will require a change in legislation it is unlikely to be before 2005 that changes will be implemented. In the meantime, overseas doctors who have passed the PLAB examination receive limited registration for the first year, which allows them to undertake supervised employment in the NHS, in either primary or secondary care. They must provide a Certificate of Selection of Employment (CSE) completed by the medical staffing officer at a hospital, or by the GP trainer where they will work, to certify that they have been selected for supervised employment in the NHS. After one year, doctors may apply to move from limited to full registration and are required to provide detailed satisfactory reports in order to do so.

Overseas trainees – permit-free training

Permit-Free Training (PFT) visas are restricted to those undertaking postgraduate medical training in the UK. They are unique to postgraduate medical education and are a means of simplifying immigration regulations for overseas trainees. Anybody without the right of abode in the UK, who would like to work here, has to apply for a work permit through their employer. New arrangements came into effect on 1 April 1997 for overseas doctors undertaking postgraduate training in a hospital or the community health services. The duration of PFT visas is now more clearly related to the training programme of the individual doctor.

To qualify for PFT in the UK an overseas doctor must satisfy the immigration authorities upon arrival in the UK of:

- their intention to undergo postgraduate training in a hospital
- their current registration or eligibility to apply for registration with the GMC (having already passed or been exempted from the PLAB test)
- their intention to leave the UK after their training
- their ability to maintain themselves and any dependants without support from public funds.

Extensions to permit-free training

The length of the extension granted depends on the type of training being pursued and the period of permit-free training already granted. Overseas doctors wishing to apply for an extension of their PFT must apply directly to the Home Office using the deanery application pack. In addition to the requirements outlined above each applicant will normally be required to show that:

- he or she will be employed or hold an acceptable appointment in a hospital or the community health services for the period of the proposed extension
- the postgraduate dean supports and recommends an extension.

The 'London Deanery Permit-Free Training – Guidelines and Extension Application Pack' has been designed to make applying for a PFT visa extension as easy as possible. It includes form PF/PGD; the Home Office will only accept originals of this form. Photocopies will not be accepted.

In London, overseas trainees requesting an extension to their PFT visa should collect a copy of this pack from their postgraduate education centre. All trainees are strongly encouraged to submit their requests for letters of support for PFT visa extensions in a timely advanced fashion. As a guide, applications should be made no less than eight weeks before the expiry date of the visa.

The following is a brief summary of the guidelines. Please note that this is a guide only: overseas trainees requesting an extension to their PFT visa should collect a copy of the 'Permit-Free Training – Guidelines and Extension Application Pack' from their postgraduate education centre as soon as possible.

Pre-registration house officer

Twelve months' PFT is allowed and this does not count towards the basic specialist or higher specialist allowance of PFT. Pre-registration house officers

(PRHOs) should apply directly to the Home Office; they do not require any recommendation from the deanery.

Basic specialist or general professional training

SHOs may be granted extensions for a period up to, but not exceeding, three years; the period spent in basic specialist training should not exceed four years in aggregate. Postgraduate deans have no discretion to recommend extensions beyond this limit. In addition the Postgraduate Dean's recommendation will normally be for a period no longer than the duration of confirmed appointment to a training post.

Higher specialist training – specialist registrar grade or equivalent: type I or type II training

Until 31 March 1997, overseas doctors were admitted to the UK provided that they intended to leave the country on completion of their training period, which could not exceed four years, except in 'exceptional' cases. This led to changes in the immigration rules from 1 April 1997, when more flexible arrangements were introduced.

The new regulations allow for entry to type I training and a Certificate of Completion of Specialist Training (CCST) for specialist registrars (SpRs) who have competed in open competition for an SpR post after 1 April 1997; the ruling cannot be applied retrospectively.

Successful applicants are entitled to extensions of PFT visas for three years in the first instance and subsequent extensions until a date six months after the achievement of the CCST, subject to satisfactory progress and assessment. These periods will be in addition to the maximum of four years available for basic professional training.

Visiting registrars on fixed-term training appointments (FTTAs) are classified as being in type II training, which does not qualify them to receive the CCST. Extensions of PFT can be supported if trainees are in a training post and can identify a specific educational goal, such as the FRCS Part III. Visiting doctors in FTTAs will be given Fixed Term Training Numbers (FTTNs).

SpRs who request an extension to their PFT visa need to collect a PFT Extension Application Pack from their postgraduate centre, complete form PF/PGD, included in the pack, and return it along with a current job appointment letter (for SpRs on type II training only) to the postgraduate dean. As with SHOs, PFT applications should be submitted in time for the forms to be processed.

Postgraduate training in general practice

In the initial discussion with the GMC about registration, doctors from any country outside the UK will be given advice about whether they can be registered or are required to take the IELTS and PLAB examinations. If they are exempt from PLAB, they can apply to the Joint Committee on Postgraduate Training for General Practice (JCPTGP) to see if any of their overseas medical experience or training can be counted towards GP training. From October 2005, the JCPTGP will be subsumed into the Postgraduate Medical Education and Training Board (PMETB).

After taking the PLAB examination, overseas-qualified doctors have to undergo three years' GP training if they want a career in general practice. No doctors who require three years' general practice training, are exempt from PLAB. Once a training rotation has been offered the doctor may apply for PFT as described above.

Who can and cannot work in NHS general practice

The regulations that say who can and who cannot work in NHS general practice are complex. European Union (EU) free movement legislation means that very many EU doctors have the right to work in the UK without further training. All they need to do is obtain GMC registration and have their EU certificate of training in general practice or of acquired rights in general practice recognised by the GMC. Any doctor who falls into this category will have a letter of confirmation from the GMC. Some doctors coming from the EU will not have this right for two reasons:

- they do not possess the necessary EU certificate
- they do possess the EU certificate but it is not recognised by the GMC because their medical degree or nationality is not from the EU.

Some of these ineligible doctors will have done some relevant training in their home country or elsewhere, which may mean they can undertake a shortened training scheme in the UK to gain a UK certificate issued by the JCPTGP. It is up to the JCPTGP to assess this training and these doctors usually need to complete some more training in the UK to be eligible for a JCPTGP certificate.

Shortened GP training

Many deaneries offer shortened GP training schemes. Shortened schemes are on offer to doctors who have undergone training for a career in specialist medicine in the UK or who have trained in relevant specialities overseas. Previous experience must be formally evaluated and accepted by the JCPTGP before acceptance on a shortened scheme can be confirmed.

The JCPTGP will collect a variety of evidence about an applicant's experience and, following the formal assessment, will inform the doctor about the amount of further training needed to be eligible for a UK Certificate of Vocational Training. As part of this process, for posts undertaken within the European Economic Area (EEA), the JCPTGP will want to know from the relevant EEA competent authority whether or not a post was approved for GP and/or specialist training in the member state. If it was approved it may be accepted in lieu of UK training.

The JCPTGP will only make a formal assessment of an applicant's experience once they have obtained full or limited registration with the GMC, or have passed Part One of the PLAB test. Doctors who are not registered with the GMC or who require the PLAB qualification and have not yet passed either of the examinations will only receive informal advice.

General practice experience and the 'accelerated route'

The JCPTGP offers certain doctors an 'accelerated route' to GP certification. Specifically, doctors who have at least five years recent experience as a GP in a family medicine system similar to the NHS or who have, in the last seven years, satisfactorily completed a family medicine training programme in a system similar to the NHS, are eligible for this route.

Doctors who are accepted onto the accelerated route have to complete a minimum of three months as a GP registrar in an approved NHS training practice. They will be formally assessed by means of the Summative Assessment Consultation Skills test and the trainer's report.

Following a quick, early assessment of doctors' eligibility for this route, based on the answers they give to a simple questionnaire, doctors are referred to the National Recruitment Office (NRO) manager, who then contacts the deanery at which the particular doctor has expressed a wish to be trained. The doctor is then interviewed by a Director of Postgraduate General Practice Education (DPGPE), who decides the amount of training required and seeks to find a post at a training practice. This is funded from Medical Postgraduate Education and Training (MPET) monies. Once the accelerated route programme has been satisfactorily completed the JCPTGP will issue a certificate of equivalent experience, which will allow that doctor to work unrestrictedly as a GP within the NHS.

EEA certificates of specific training and of acquired rights

EU law defines in very broad terms the length and content of GP training in every member state. Member states are required only to issue certificates of specific training (CSTs) in general practice to doctors who have undertaken the EU-defined programme.

An employer can be relatively confident that a doctor who has an EU CST has been trained in general practice up to a minimum level.

However, all member states are also allowed to define what is known as 'acquired rights' doctors. There are a multitude of acquired rights categories and we know that some doctors from the EU who have acquired rights to work as a GP principal in the NHS have no training or experience as a GP. Notwithstanding their legal right to work, there is, of course, no legal requirement on an employer to employ them if they do not think that their experience is adequate.

Doctors who have a CST of a certificate of acquired rights from another member state invariably have to apply to the GMC for confirmation of their eligibility to work as a GP within the NHS. The management services of the GMC scrutinises their EU certificates and will confirm or not that the doctor is exempt from the need to obtain a JCPTGP certificate and can work in the UK. A letter is issued stating the doctor has a legal right to work as a GP in the UK.

If the GMC confirms that a doctor is not exempt from the need to hold a UK vocational training certificate an application will need to be made to the JCPTGP for an independent assessment of the applicant's experience and doctors are advised in writing what further training is necessary to obtain a certificate of equivalent experience to enable them to work in the UK.

Figure 12.1 offers a summary of the process.

Supporting overseas and refugee doctors into training

Clinical attachments

Clinical attachments are necessary for overseas doctors to understand the NHS and to obtain the references to apply for SHO posts. There are two types of clinical attachments needed and the London Deanery is involved in offering both types.[2]

- Induction and short exposure to a speciality (two to four weeks). Overseas doctors with a visitor's visa, wanting to move from recent working in their own country to being employed in the UK.
- Supported clinical attachment programmes for overseas and refugee doctors who have been out of medicine for some years. These doctors require induction, an understanding of the NHS or primary and secondary care, exposure to clinical situations as observers, opportunities to practise history-taking and examination skills, and teaching in communication skills.

Regulations for EEA doctors requesting recognition as GPs legally entitled
to work in the UK

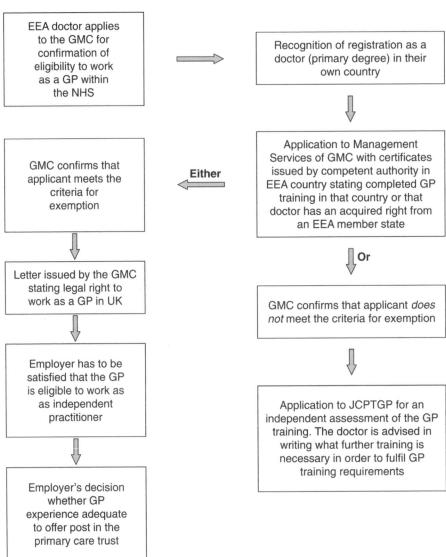

Figure 12.1   Regulations for EEA doctors requesting recognition as GPs legally entitled to
work in the UK.

In 2003 a pan-London scheme was set up for 'job ready' refugee doctors. The
aims were to:

● expand the concept from traditional one-to-one clinical attachments to cohort attachments for five to six doctors in a network of participating trusts

- introduce new clinical concepts of a core curriculum, supervision by a refugee project tutor, exposure to more than one speciality and to the interface between primary care and hospital medicine in a three-month attachment
- evaluate effectiveness by feedback from tutors and doctors and by monitoring the number of doctors who achieved substantive jobs
- identify factors that contribute to success in obtaining jobs
- assess the transferability of the scheme to other trusts as an ongoing training opportunity.

At the end of the scheme, over half of the participating refugee doctors gained posts in open competition. The majority reported that the scheme increased their self-esteem as refugee doctors. Unfortunately, as only a small group of 29 doctors were involved, no individual factors associated with success in getting a job could be identified. From the evaluation forms and discussion at meetings it was possible, however, to identify what the participants and tutors found useful, which included the placement in cohorts, regular tutorials covering a curriculum, exposure to more than one speciality and the ability of tutors to write realistic references. Doctors favoured receiving these references too as their UK references. It has not been possible yet to assess transferability of the scheme as an ongoing training opportunity.[3]

The GP department of the London Deanery runs the 'Clinical Experience Scheme for Overseas and Refugee Doctors', which started in April 2003. This offers a two-day induction course, then two clinical attachments – the first six weeks in a general practice followed by six weeks in a hospital department. During the 12-week scheme there is a half-day release run by GPs and the IELTS is provided for further language development and communication skills. Fifty-six doctors have now completed the scheme and 24 of them now have posts, of which nine have been successful in obtaining three-year GP training rotations.

Supernumerary posts for refugee doctors

Despite undertaking structured clinical attachments, many refugee doctors will not have practised medicine for a few years. The London Deanery has organised a new scheme of supernumerary posts to enable these doctors to experience 'hands on' medicine in the UK. The 'Placing Refugee doctors In Medical Employment' (PRIME) project places job-ready refugee doctors, who have undertaken a clinical attachment with a satisfactory report from the supervising consultant, in supernumerary SHO posts for six months in the speciality of their choice. Two acute hospital trusts and a mental health trust are involved in the scheme, which allows doctors to be placed in cohorts, thus enabling group learning and support and supervision by a project tutor. A database has been established of refugee doctor supernumerary post-holders charting their career progression.

Refugee doctor general practice vocational training rotations

Developing protected three-year GP training rotations for refugee doctors is one element in the GP recruitment strategy of the London Deanery. These are all projects of the London Deanery, and are advertised separately from the national recruitment of general practice vocational training scheme (GPVTS) trainees. However, the same recruitment process and criteria are applied, as for other VTS placements in the deanery, to maintain consistency, quality and standards.

Because of the specific needs of these doctors, the rotation is 18 months in hospital and 18 months in general practice. The SHO posts are chosen from:

- geriatric medicine: this post is essential, as these doctors have no equivalent in their countries of origin and we need to make sure that they are both competent in general medicine and taught the skills of dealing with elderly people
- obstetrics and gynaecology
- paediatrics
- psychiatry.

All proposed SHO posts are supernumerary and in departments that already have educational approval for GP training. The experience, education and training provided by these posts will be oriented towards the individual learning needs of the refugee doctors. For the first and second months the refugee doctors are 'protected' and assessed by their consultants for competence to work independently as SHOs. The refugee doctors attend the GP VTS half-day release.[4]

Refugee doctor GP rotations have been set up at St Mary's Hospital (north-west London), Homerton and Whipps Cross Hospitals (north-east London) and Barnet and Chase Farm hospitals (north-central London). Further funding has been obtained to set up two more rotations in the north-central sector, at The Whittington Hospital and the North Middlesex Hospital. Each rotation is for three doctors and started in August 2004.

International recruitment

London EU GP international recruitment

Many primary care trusts (PCTs) in London identified international recruitment as an integral part of their recruitment strategy. The Department of Health has supported nationwide initiatives and it has been working with the pan-London Action Group (PLAG) to provide expertise and funding. North-east, north-central and north-west London strategic health authorities (SHAs) have worked collaboratively with the London Deanery and the Centre for General Practice and

Primary Care at Queen Mary College, University of London, to develop an induction programme for EU GPs. The aim of the programme is to prepare EU GPs for working with primary care teams in London and to facilitate their successful integration into general practice.

There were two recruitment visits in 2003, to Paris and Madrid, and one in 2004 to Poland. During the visits the recruitment teams described general practice in London and talked about the PCTs that were offering posts. The London Deanery team interviewed the EU GPs and they had a verbal language assessment.

Suitable candidates were invited to London to a pre-assessment weekend. During this time they visited practices and had discussions with GPs and PCT leads. Attention was given to the EU doctors need for housing and other aspects of settling in a foreign country. The London Deanery organised an observed simulated clinical examination (OSCE), and the language assessors undertook further written and aural language assessments.

In September 2003, 10 EU GPs formed the pilot group for the first EU GP induction programme for London. Below is a description of this induction programme and the changes that have taken place to it following evaluation. Advice was taken from a previous development of an EU induction programme for south-east London.[5]

There are five elements of the EU GP induction programme, as follows.

Core sessions

The core sessions were held at the Centre for General Practice and Primary Care, Queen Mary College, University of London. Topics covered were: working with hospitals; community services; understanding London patients (working in a multiracial society); prescribing; clinical governance; psychiatry; national service frameworks (NSFs); alcohol and drug abuse; guidelines and protocols; child health; and terminal care services.

Language support sessions

The English language sessions had two components: basic English and medical English, so improving communication skills.

Practice-based sessions

Each EU GP was placed in a practice with an EU GP mentor. The preference was that this should be a training practice, but in some of the PCTs that were offering posts there are few training practices. So other practices were chosen, in which there was some experience of education and teaching, and were assessed to be an appropriate learning environment. The clinical experience in the practice was to enable the EU GP to understand how UK general practice is organised, to understand the roles and responsibilities for the primary healthcare teams, and to further develop the EU GP's communication and consulting skills (Table 12.1 and Table 12.2).

Table 12.1: Clinical experience in the practice

How general practice is organised:
- patient access
- referrals
- community in the hospital
- practice records and computers
- visits
- out-of-hours
- prescribing
- audit

Roles and responsibilities of different members of the primary healthcare team (PHCT)

To understand community services

To further develop communication and consulting skills

Table 12. 2: Methods of learning in the practice

GP mentor

Involvement of whole PHCT

Agreed educational plan

Formative learning needs assessment: OSCEs, confidence rating scale, multiple-choice questionnaires

Joint surgeries

Debrief after surgeries

Tutorials

NHS Logbook

Outpatient Department sessions

Certain areas (such as paediatrics and gynaecology) are known not to be the responsibility of some EU GPs and therefore time was given to help the clinical skills and knowledge in these areas.

Peer support and communication skills sessions

The ethos of this half-day was learner-centred education, with an emphasis on attitude and encouraging shared feelings and peer support. It was problem-based learning and was intended to encourage the EU GP to be a part of the primary healthcare team.

Issues raised

The greatest problem during the induction period was the lack of appropriate GMC registration and therefore the doctors not being on the supplementary list. This meant that they could not work as independent practitioners and this caused frustration for the EU mentor and GPs, as well as a regression of some of their learning. Some of the EU GPs' command of English, written and spoken, was not adequate for consultations.

As a result seven of the 10 EU GPs were granted extensions of up to three months. This was either to improve their English or (once their certificates were authenticated by the GMC and they were on the supplementary list) to enable them to work independently with their mentor. One EU GP's practice experience was extended due to maternity leave.

Following the evaluation of the first programme a number of changes were agreed:

- future programmes based in London will last for 20 weeks (not 12 weeks)
- although all EU GPs have a right to work in the UK there is a selection process to join the programme
- the necessary registrations, GMC and supplementary list are required before EU GPs are accepted on the induction programme
- EU GPs must have the equivalent of IELTS 6.5 before joining the programme
- one month's intensive English tuition at the beginning of the induction programme
- there is a greater appreciation of the practice experience and the role of the mentor, so the GP experience is in blocks of days
- allow the EU GPs to choose their employing practices during the induction programme
- reinstate the importance of recruitment lead at PCT level
- all involved in international recruitment to understand the process recommended for London: to enable this an international recruitment handbook for GP recruitment has been written.[6]

New consultant entry scheme

For many different reasons, some SpRs do not immediately take up a substantive consultant post after completing their training. Following collaboration between the Department of Health, the postgraduate deaneries, the workforce development confederations and NHS professionals, two pilot studies were established in London and Essex, and Manchester and Cumbria.

The aim of the New Consultant Entry Scheme (NCES) was to facilitate recently qualified specialists to undertake a fixed-term consultant appointment of six to 12 months. This appointment allows new consultants not to be committed to a post or area for longer than a year, and it also provides new consultants with a mentor and an extra two sessions (professional activities) per week for continuing professional development (CPD). The posts were provided by an NHS trust and comprised vacancies that may not have previously been filled for a variety of reasons, or because there may only be short-term funding available and therefore the trusts could not commit themselves to appointing a consultant for more than a year. It also provides the trust with evidence that the post may or may not be needed for its future clinical service.

The new consultants are employed by NHS Professionals, a special health authority, with the normal terms and conditions of service expected from all consultants working within the NHS. NHS Professionals charges a fee of 7.5% of the consultant's basic salary and this is paid either by the Workforce Development Confederation or the individual trust.

The pilot studies ran from autumn 2003 until spring 2004 when, following further discussions with interested parties, the NCES was rolled out nationally.

There are benefits for the consultants:

- it is a proper consultant post and is not a locum or 'junior' consultant
- experience of being a consultant without any long-term commitment
- have a mentor appointed
- have two sessions for CPD
- do not have difficulty with locums
- terms and conditions are agreed
- a worthwhile job whilst waiting for a permanent post
- good on the doctor's curriculum vitae.

There are also benefits for the trust involved:

- has a consultant whilst waiting for a permanent appointment
- does not need College approval
- may only have short-term funding
- locums may be variable
- counts towards Government consultant targets.

To contact NHS Professionals for more information use the doctors helpline: +44 0114 290 2647.

Summary

The numbers of doctors working in the NHS continues to rise, and doctors are recruited from both UK graduates and abroad. It is essential that patients have confidence in their doctor, and the medical team, and only by setting and applying standards can this be achieved.

References

1 www.ielts.org

2 Kiernan P and Trafford P (2004) Refugee doctor GP VTS rotations. In: Jackson N and Carter Y (eds) *Refugee Doctors: support, development and integration in the NHS*. Radcliffe Publishing, Oxford; 131–46.

3 Ong Y L and Gayen A (2003) Helping refugee doctors get their first jobs: the pan-London clinical attachment scheme. *Hospital Medicine* **64**: 488–90.

4 Ong Y L and Trafford P (2004) Clinical attachments in primary and secondary care. In: Jackson N and Carter Y (eds) *Refugee Doctors: support, development and integration in the NHS*. Radcliffe Publishing, Oxford; 117–29.

5 Essex B (2001) South East London EU GP Induction programme. Locally published report.

6 Delacourt L and Heatley R (2004) *Handbook for EU GP Recruitment*. NC/NEL International Recruitment Management Board, London.

CHAPTER 13

Return to medicine

Anne Hastie and Timothy Peters

Introduction

The recruitment and retention of GPs and hospital consultants has become a national priority. *The NHS Plan*[1] required the appointment of an additional 2 000 general practitioners (GPs) and 7 000 consultants into substantive posts by 2004. One of the most cost-effective methods of increasing the number of GPs and consultants in the workforce is to recruit doctors who have not been working for a variety of reasons.

The GP returner scheme

In November 2002 the Department of Health launched a 'National Returner Campaign', which included the introduction in England of the 'GP Returner Scheme'[2] to facilitate a re-entry programme through refresher training. The campaign was aimed at qualified GPs in the following circumstances:

- working as locums rather than in substantive NHS posts
- who are not working
- who are working but not in general practice.

Recruitment

At the beginning of the campaign, adverts were placed in national newspapers and medical press, including the telephone number of the Returners Hotline (0845 606 0345) operated by NHS Professionals. This is an agency, based in Sheffield, which provides an administrative function for the scheme on behalf of the Department of Health. Doctors interested in returning to general practice are directed to their local postgraduate deanery where they are invited for an informal interview to discuss their individual circumstances. Deaneries only had a very small number of doctors returning to general practice each year before the introduction of the GP Returner Scheme when numbers increased tenfold and applications are continuing at a steady pace. It is probable that the increasing emphasis on flexible working has attracted some of these doctors, who left because of the previous rigidity of employment within medicine,[3] back to the NHS.

Situation at the time of application

GPs considering returning to general practice have a variety of backgrounds, with no single group dominating. The most common situations at the time of application include:

- family commitments
- working abroad
- medical management
- health problems
- pharmaceutical industry
- other medical specialities
- journalism
- retired.

Some doctors left general practice for new careers thinking the grass would be greener but after a number of years discovered this was not the case and general practice looked the more attractive option.

Eligibility

Not all doctors are eligible to join the GP Returner Scheme because of current legislation. The Committee of General Practice Education Directors (COGPED) provided the following guidance on the entry criteria for doctors wishing to join the scheme.

- The doctor must be eligible to work in general practice and evidence should be submitted to the deanery.
- They should normally have worked as a GP in the UK or British armed services for at least one year (including as a GP registrar).
- They would not normally be offered refresher training if they had been working in a substantive NHS GP post during the previous 24 months. (There may be circumstances when refresher training is appropriate following shorter periods.)
- The returner should normally work at least half-time during the period of refresher training, including clinical and educational activities. Exceptions can be made in individual cases at the discretion of the Director of Postgraduate General Practice Education (DPGPE).

- They must agree to refresh their skills in dealing with GP emergencies.
- They should not work as GP locums during their period of refresher training.
- Returners may work in another field of medicine or in a non-medical career at the discretion of the DPGPE while undergoing refresher training.
- They should indicate their intention to work in a substantive NHS GP post for at least two years (or the equivalent part-time) following their refresher training. This may not necessarily all be completed immediately following refresher training, for example maternity leave.
- Approval to join the returner scheme is subject to finding a suitable placement.
- Approval is also subject to:
  - acceptance on to the performer list of the primary care trust (PCT)
  - occupational health clearance
  - screening by the Disclosure Services of the Criminal Records Bureau.

A regulatory framework exists, which stipulates those doctors who are eligible to work in general practice. The most recent regulations came into force on 30 January 1998, as a result of The National Health Service (Vocational Training for General Medical Practice) Regulations 1997. Doctors are eligible to work in general practice in the UK[4] in the following circumstances:

- hold a Joint Committee on Postgraduate Training for General Practice (JCPTGP) certificate of prescribed or equivalent experience
- have a legal exemption to holding a JCPTGP certificate
- have acquired rights to work in general practice (in some circumstances this only enables the doctor to work as a locum or salaried GP).

Placement

The GP Returner Scheme allows a period of refresher training of up to six months full-time or 12 months part-time. This is usually undertaken in a training practice, although the DPGPE can approve placements in other practices with suitable educational support. For most returners it takes between three and nine months from initial contact to the beginning of refresher training, for a variety of reasons. It may be difficult to find a placement for some doctors, whereas others take time before they feel able to make the commitment.

The content of the refresher training, based on a learning needs assessment, varies from one returner to another. For instance a returner who has been working abroad in general practice may be up to date clinically, but may need a period of reorientation to the NHS. In contrast, a doctor who has not been working for 10 years because of domestic commitments will need updating in current clinical practice as well as administrative aspects, including the use of IT in primary care. There have been many changes in primary care over the last decade with an increasingly multiprofessional approach.[5] Exposure and an understanding of working in a primary healthcare team is particularly important for those doctors who have not worked in general practice for many years.

GP returners are employed in a similar way to GP registrars with the practice paying their salary, which is reimbursed by the deanery through their PCT. In addition, the educational supervisor receives the equivalent of a trainer's grant and returners receive a payment towards their professional expenses. Many of the doctors returning to general practice are eligible for payment under the 'NHS GP Golden Hello' scheme.[6]

Assessment

Each doctor has very different refresher training requirements, and assessments need to be tailored to individual returners. Some doctors will feel very vulnerable so the timing of assessments needs to be carefully planned and it is essential the returner and trainer keep documentation of all assessments. The following guidance is recommended for the assessment of GP returners.

- A self-assessment package should be used prior to organising a refresher training placement. In addition, a knowledge test, such as a multiple-choice questionnaire (MCQ), based on the Summative Assessment MCQ or a PEP-2000 (PEP-2000 can be ordered through www.rcgp-scotland.org.uk, click on to 'life-long learning') may be helpful. The results of this initial assessment should be used to inform the deanery representative on the type and length of refresher training required.
- Formative assessment by the trainer:
  - PEP-2000 is recommended for all cases but the timing should be agreed between the trainer and returner; only sections relevant to the returner's planned employment exit strategy need be completed but should include clinical components
  - other assessment methods, tailored to the individual trainer and returner, should be used at regular intervals throughout the period of refresher training; trainers may wish to use the same tools as they use for their GP registrars
  - returners should complete (as a method of formative assessment) at least one and preferably all three of the Summative Assessment consulting skills, written component and MCQ.
- A structured trainer's report should be completed, signed and returned to the DPGPE (or the deanery representative) for each returner within one month of the planned finishing date.

It is recognised that some doctors may require rather more rigorous assessment than described in this guidance, and the trainer should be guided by the DPGPE (or the deanery representative). If difficulties are identified during the period of the refresher training, help should be sort from the deanery as soon as possible.

Exit strategy

The initial interview with returners, prior to placement, should identify an exit strategy, which may need to involve the local PCT. The refresher training needs to take into account the type of employment doctors are planning for their future. If they want to work exclusively as a GP assistant they may not need to include practice administration but this would be important for someone hoping to become a GP partner. Peer support for returners is important and the deanery is in a position to co-ordinate a peer support network. At the end of the period of refresher training doctors may require further support, and this can be provided through various activities, including mentoring and self-directed learning groups.

An exit interview with the DPGPE or their representative is helpful and gives the deanery feedback on the scheme with suggestions for improvement. In addition, interviewers should discuss with returners their future career intentions, educational needs and other issues. Comments from those who have already finished the scheme have been overwhelmingly positive and include:

'Confidence boosting'
'Supported in what I wanted to do'
'Getting back to work in a protected environment'
'Excellent resources and information about the scheme'
'Equipped to move back into general practice'
'Support was there when I needed it.'

The hospital returner scheme

As part of the overall strategy to increase the numbers of hospital consultants by 7000, as required by *The NHS Plan*,[1] a scheme to encourage former hospital doctors to return to clinical practice has been developed. During 2000 a pilot scheme was operated by the former North and South Thames deaneries.

London pilot returner scheme

There was variable anecdotal evidence of doctors who had left the NHS, mainly in training grades, but who were interested in returning to clinical practice. A pilot scheme of 20 placements was initiated and advertised by 'snow-balling' throughout the region. More extensive advertising was not used as the demand was uncertain and funds were limited. The criteria for entry to the pilot scheme were relatively restrictive because of the limited funds available.

The majority of trainees were at SHO grade and two were at SpR grade. The average time out of clinical practice was seven years, with a range of three to 15 years. The reasons for not working were predominantly domestic commitments but absence overseas, chronic ill-health, full-time research posts and a variety of individual reasons also contributed. Approximately one-quarter of trainees chose to train in the shortage specialities of general practice, psychiatry, paediatrics and histopathology. Professional assessment and advice was obtained from the appropriate lead consultant for flexible training, and most applicants on the pilot scheme were placed in teaching hospitals. Placements were for one year, renewable, and most doctors have either returned to training (usually in a flexible training capacity) or have obtained substantive (consultant, associate specialist, staff grade) posts within the NHS. Overall, the pilot scheme has been considered a success because it returned doctors to clinical practice, who would have otherwise been lost to the profession. Current participants have been transferred to the 'Flexible Career Scheme Returner Programme' administered by NHS Professionals

Hospital flexible careers scheme

Following the successful London pilot scheme, a national (England and Wales, but excluding Scotland and Northern Ireland) returner scheme was launched and is administered by NHS Professionals. The scheme is called the 'Flexible Career Scheme Returner Programme' and should not be confused with the 'GP Flexible Career Scheme', which is described in Chapter 14. There have been several national and local advertising campaigns encouraging hospital doctors to return to clinical practice. Doctors who are accepted to the Flexible Career Scheme Returner Programme work in a supernumerary capacity.

Recruitment

Referrals of potential returners come from a variety of sources with many responding to the advertising campaigns and articles in the medical and general press. Returners contact NHS Professionals in Sheffield and after preliminary screening for suitability are referred to deanery contacts for further advice and processing. Other potential returners come from a variety of sources, including word of mouth, self-referrals, local postgraduate deans, local trusts and doctors approaching deanery colleagues for career counselling.

The first step is to determine eligibility for the scheme. These have recently been reviewed and are currently:

- to have been out of a training programme or active NHS clinical practice for at least two years
- hold full GMC registration
- have permanent right of residence (refugee, immigrant and overseas doctors)

- have realistic aims and objectives and to be able to benefit from the scheme.

The Flexible Career Scheme Returner Programme is not appropriate for doctors who have been (repeatedly) unsuccessful in applying for training posts, for doctors wishing to retrain in another speciality and for those with conditional registration from the GMC.

The scheme should not be confused with the long-standing Flexible Training Scheme for junior doctors, although some deaneries have been using the Flexible Career Scheme Retainer Scheme as a way of supporting doctors whilst they are on a waiting list for flexible training funding. The Flexible Career Scheme Returner Programme is distinct from the Flexible Career Scheme Retainer Scheme, although both are administered by NHS Professionals under the Flexible Career Scheme umbrella.

Procedures

Following enquiries about the Flexible Career Scheme Returner Programme, doctors are invited to contact their local deanery for interview and discussions with the appropriate associate dean. The basic aims and eligibility criteria are explained and detailed planning is undertaken, if appropriate. The Part 1 application form is completed and signed by both the doctor and the associate dean. A contribution of £700 is payable to the doctor for professional expenses and up to £1000 is available for study leave programmes. The scheme does not provide full training for doctors to reach their long-term objectives, for example consultant, GP, associate specialist, but it does facilitate their return to clinical practice so that they are eligible and (hopefully) successful in applying for posts in open competition, for example SHO, SpR, in their chosen speciality. Doctors who have already obtained their Certificate of Completion of Specialist Training (CCST) in an appropriate speciality will be assisted to re-skill and will, it is hoped, be successful in applying for a consultant post.

Most returners express a desire to return to part-time clinical practice. Although doctors are encouraged to work full-time in their first placement if possible, at least six sessions a week is generally considered the minimum. A measure of their commitment, the need for a minimum intensity of learning and financial considerations determines this requirement.

General practice training

It is important that the doctors have realistic aims and objectives. Many doctors believe that general practice is a simple option, but they need to understand the amount of training that is necessary and the structure of the training programme. It may well be that their previous SHO posts have 'lapsed' during their period out of clinical medicine and a full two years of appropriate hospital SHO posts are necessary. The DPGPE should be consulted at an early stage in the process, and a period of attachment to a practice may be advisable for doctors who have no experience in general practice and are unaware of the recent developments in primary care.

Under ideal conditions the successful completion of a six-month Flexible Career Scheme SHO placement is followed by a successful application to a GP vocational training scheme (VTS). Consideration needs to be given as to the most preferable initial SHO placement if a returner wants to train for general practice. Care of the elderly (geriatrics) and accident and emergency are proving to be very suitable for both future GPs and hospital doctors returning to clinical medicine after prolonged periods.

Currently, approximately 15% of hospital returners are planning a career in general practice. For some doctors, whose previous training was reasonably advanced (for example three to five years) the FCS returner placement can be approved by the speciality royal college and the Royal College of General Practice (RCGP) as part of their GP training requirements. Some potential GP trainees may need a placement in a supernumerary pre-registration house officer (PRHO) post or even need to attend some final-year undergraduate courses.

To date, several of the initial 15 potential GP trainees have obtained GPVTS placements, but longer term follow-up will be necessary to gauge the overall value of the programme in returning doctors for general practice training and to optimise the retraining pathway.

Pre-registration house officer returners

A limited number of doctors left the profession immediately after graduation and for a variety of reasons, including disillusionment, ill-health or moving abroad, did not complete one or more PRHO placements. These doctors are therefore only eligible for the provisional registration with the GMC. Returning to clinical practice at this level, particularly after a prolonged period of absence, may not be a realistic objective. The on-call commitments are particularly challenging, although the European Working Time Directive (EWTD) and the proposed new foundation programmes will make these less daunting. To date only a small number of doctors have rejoined the NHS at this level.

Senior House Officer returners

Apart from doctors who have previously held consultant or (senior) registrar placements, this is the level at which most returners will enter. Funding is available for six months' full-time training or up to 12 months pro-rata part-time. Extensions are not normally allowed so it is important that only doctors who are likely to gain a substantive post in open competition on leaving the scheme, are accepted.

Specialist registrars

Doctors who have reached the registrar grade in their chosen speciality, and who have obtained one or more postgraduate qualifications, are relatively easy to place under the scheme. The level to which previous training has been reached is much more important than the length of time out of practice in determining the ease of re-entry. After six months' retaining most returner SpRs can gain entry to the normal training programmes, obtaining a national training number (NTN) in open competition. The difficulty reflects the overall competitiveness in a particular speciality and to date many returners have opted for shortage specialities, such as psychiatry, paediatrics and pathology.

Consultants

A small number of established consultants (approximately 10) have applied to join the scheme. These are usually colleagues who have been seconded to senior administrative posts in the NHS, medical royal college, etc., and who would wish to return to clinical practice. Some are doctors who have been operating solely within the private sector and wish to return to the NHS. A number of doctors who have taken early retirement have expressed an interest in the scheme but to date none in London have successfully returned to worthwhile NHS practice.

Returning consultants usually plan to work part-time and wish to avoid onerous on-call or on-take commitments. They do, however, contribute to the service commitments and can usually be suitably placed. Many have valuable transferable skills, for example medico-legal qualifications, experience in the pharmaceutical industry and academic (including deanery) experience.

Placement

Obtaining suitable placements for returning doctors may prove difficult. The advice of the DPGPE, the lead consultants for flexible training in the appropriate speciality or the patch associate dean are particularly valuable. Major teaching hospitals are often inappropriate venues. Personal contacts and district general hospitals with a special interest and expertise in assisting these doctors are usually the best way forward. It should be emphasised that although the doctor's salary is fully funded there are significant opportunity costs, including the need for careful supervision with additional training and mentoring requirements. It is usually a few months before the doctor can function at an appropriate level, such as undertaking on-call commitments.

Doctors are employed by the trusts under their usual terms and conditions of service and returning doctors cannot be imposed on a trust against the trust's wishes. A successful placement as an unpaid clinical assistant is a useful prelude to being offered a supernumerary SHO post by the same trust. There is, however, no guarantee from either the deanery or NHS Professionals that a placement will be found. Approximately 5% of doctors eligible to join the scheme do not proceed to find a post and leave the scheme voluntarily.

When a suitable placement has been agreed a detailed Part 2 FCS Returners Form is completed. This indicates an agreed timetable, a personal learning plan with agreed objectives and measures as well as a section for completion by the trust's human resources department. An identified appraiser and appropriate dates are noted and the clinical tutor or programme director countersigns the form. Final approval by the deanery is necessary before submission to NHS Professionals, who negotiate salary scales and starting dates with the trust.

Conclusions

The GP returner scheme is proving to be a greater success than originally anticipated and will make a significant increase to the number of GPs working. The scheme provides a supportive environment for returners to refresh their skills and ensures the quality of their work through a formative assessment process.

The hospital doctor's returner scheme has been in place in the London Deanery and adjoining deaneries for approximately five years. Well over 200 applications have been processed and results to date are encouraging, with the numbers of applications continuing to increase. All but a few doctors who have joined the scheme have returned to active and productive clinical practice, although some have decided largely due to the changes in clinical practice and NHS working, etc., not to proceed.

References

1 Secretary of State for Health (2000) *The NHS Plan – A Plan for Investment, A Plan for Reform.* Department of Health, London.

2 Department of Health (2002) *General Practitioners – Returning to the NHS.* Department of Health, London.

3 Vaughan C (1995) Career choices for Generation X. Young doctors want flexible career paths, not long term commitments. *BMJ.* **311**: 525–6.

4 . Joint Committee on Postgraduate General Practice Training for General Practice (2002) *A Guide to Certification.* JCPTGP, London.

5 Secretary of State for Health (1997) *The New NHS.* HMSO, London.

6 www.doh.gov.uk/pricare/goldenhello

CHAPTER 14

Educational schemes to retain qualified general practitioners

Anne Hastie and Rebecca Viney

Introduction

The history of higher professions, including medicine, has been one of male domination[1] but in theory women now have equal access to senior posts, although elements of inequality still exist. In general practice nearly one-third of doctors undertake professional duties as freelance and salaried general practitioners (GPs) (previously known as non-principals), including those on the GP Retainer Scheme and Flexible Career Scheme. More than 70% of salaried and freelance GPs are female.[2]

There have been long-standing concerns about medical workforce planning, which is complex and has had a fragmented approach in the past.[3] It takes a minimum of four years to train a newly qualified doctor as a GP, and many GPs choose to work less than full-time or stop working for a period of time because of domestic commitments. Allen[4] found that only 5% of women doctors were not working, but 36% were working less than full-time compared with only 2% of male doctors. In 1998, Lambert and Goldacre[5] raised concerns about the number of Whole Time Equivalents (WTE) available for work in general practice because they found that 53% of women were working part-time.

The White Paper *The New NHS*[6] puts an emphasis on primary care, because it is usually patients' first point of contact, and the GP acts as gatekeeper to the rest of the NHS. Improving standards through clinical governance receives priority and requires appropriate education and training of all those working in primary care.

The development of the GP Retainer Scheme in 1998,[7] followed by the Flexible Career Scheme in 2002,[8] with the emphasis on education and supervision, were seen as a contribution to improving the recruitment and retention of GPs as well as facilitating the future uptake of senior roles in primary care by more female GPs.

The GP retainer scheme

The 'Doctors' Retainer Scheme' was introduced in 1969 to allow doctors aged under 55 years, who were unable to practise full-time for personal reasons, an opportunity to do a limited amount of paid professional work in order to maintain some exposure to clinical medicine. The scheme was originally introduced with hospital doctors in mind but became more popular in general practice, because the employing practice received an allowance towards the salary of the retainee.[9] In 1991, a working party on women doctors and their careers[10] highlighted a steady rise in those joining the Doctors' Retainer Scheme, with 90% working in general practice. Although the working party acknowledged limitations of the scheme, in particular the restriction of working for a maximum two sessions per week and the lack of educational support, it failed to recommend any changes.

By June 1998, after detailed discussion between the British Medical Association (BMA) and the Department of Health, the GP Retainer Scheme was introduced.[7] The new scheme was designed to ensure that doctors who could only undertake a small amount of paid professional work kept in touch with general practice, in order to retain their skills and progress their careers, with a view to returning to a substantive NHS general practice post in the future. The scheme includes clinical and educational components, offering retainees an opportunity to do a small amount of paid professional work combined with involvement in postgraduate medical education sessions.

The GP Retainer Scheme is open to any GP who has a Joint Committee on Postgraduate Training for General Practice (JCPTGP) certificate or is able to demonstrate acquired rights[11] and intends to return to a career in general practice. The scheme is not intended for those committed to a career in another sector, such as GP academics. Retainees usually have well-founded personal reasons for undertaking only limited paid employment and the Director of Postgraduate General Practice Education (DPGPE) will be expected to take individual circumstances into account when deciding whether to accept a doctor to the scheme.

An average of four sessions per week, up to a maximum of 52 sessions per quarter, can be worked and the minimum number of sessions per week is one, except during annual or study leave. Doctors who join the scheme work in practices where they receive regular support and input from a named GP(s), who acts as their educational facilitator and clinical supervisor. The role of the retainee is supernumerary but the practice benefits from the input of a well-motivated doctor who keeps up to date with current practice. The practice receives a sessional payment towards the cost of employing the retainee and retainees receive £310 per annum towards their professional expenses. The practice should be able to offer the retainee a full range of general medical services in a modern general practice setting, including home visits.

Practice approval for the GP Retainer Scheme

Any practice, general medical services (GMS) or personal medical services (PMS), can be approved for employing retainees if it can demonstrate that it is working towards core criteria similar to the JCPTGP's minimum educational criteria for training practices, over an agreed timescale (*see* modified Joint Committee criteria below). Postgraduate training practices will automatically meet the criteria.

Modified Joint Committee criteria

Below are the ideal criteria that practices should aim towards; however, good evidence of steady progress towards these goals will be sufficient in many cases.

- All medical records and hospital correspondence must be filed in practice notes, in chronological order.
- Records must contain easily discernible drug therapy lists for patients on long-term therapy.
- Eighty per cent of summaries in medical records – practices must be making progress towards these targets. Slow progress in otherwise satisfactory practices should lead to a shorter period of reselection than the deanery norm.
- All practices must have methods for monitoring prescribing habits as part of audit, and should have a practice formulary or a prescribing list, with a policy on how the list is reviewed and implemented.
- All practices must have a library of books and journals (this can be online).

Education

All GPs on the scheme need to demonstrate they have undertaken continuing professional development (CPD) and produce a personal development plan (PDP). Retainees undertake 28 hours of paid education annually, and three hours of this includes educational supervision within the practice. A named GP who works regularly within the practice (not necessarily a partner) is appointed as the retainee's educational facilitator and a named GP (not necessarily the educational facilitator) is appointed as clinical supervisor. The clinical supervisor should be available to provide help and advice during sessions, and at the end of the session to debrief, discuss dilemmas and interesting cases if required.

Induction

When joining a practice, the newly appointed retainee should be provided with a practice information pack and an induction programme. Information should include times and dates of practice meetings, current practice audit and in-house educational programmes. A set of practice protocols with details of any healthcare improvement programme initiatives should be provided, with instruction in the use of any appropriate template entries. A copy of the practice formulary should also be provided, with an explanation of current prescribing aims and information about members of the primary healthcare team and their areas of expertise.

The role of the educational facilitator

Protected time should be made available for both facilitators and retainees to meet on a regular basis, at a mutually convenient time, for tutorials, feedback, case discussion and other aspects of general practice that retainees feel are needed. Retainees must formulate a personal development plan designed to review their previous year's work, set learning objectives for the coming year and have an opportunity to discuss their career progress and future plans. The practice Educational Facilitator advises on the educational provisions for retainees and facilitates the identification of personal learning needs.

Time on the scheme

The length of time a doctor can be on the GP Retainer Scheme is usually five years and there is no age limit to joining the scheme, providing there is an intention to return to a career in general practice. Family commitments are by far the most frequent reason given for joining the GP Retainer Scheme and the five-year time limit is very unpopular. Retainees comment that it takes longer than five years before the youngest child reaches school age,[12] but it could also be argued that the five-year time limit does give some protection against producing a long-term ghetto for women GPs. In individual circumstances, and at the discretion of the DPGPE, the scheme may be extended to a maximum of 10 years, and maternity leave is not part of this time.

The GP Flexible Career Scheme

On 29 November 2002, the Department of Health launched the Flexible Career Scheme (FCS) for GPs, with the aim of providing additional supported part-time posts for GPs.[8] The scheme was implemented in response to the recruitment and retention crisis in general practice,[13] the NHS *Improving Working Lives Standard*[14] and new national legislation to provide flexible and family friendly employment.[15]

The Flexible Career Scheme aims to demonstrate that part-time working can be a valuable asset to both individual doctors and practices. It enables GPs to strike the right balance between their work and home lives in an educational environment. In this way it helps to support GPs who might otherwise leave the profession because they are unable to find posts that meet their particular needs, and it may also encourage GPs who have retired or left general practice to return. Doctors on the scheme work in a substantive capacity.

Eligibility to join the Flexible Career Scheme

The Flexible Career Scheme is open to GPs, regardless of age, who wish to work between two and five sessions per week as a salaried GP in an educationally supported post. Sessions can be 'annualised' to allow greater flexibility if desired (104–260 sessions per year). GPs may want to work part-time for a variety of reasons; for example, they may be a carer, a portfolio GP, an academic, wish to have a career break or downsize near retirement.[16] Sessions can be annualised to suit doctors' individual needs, enabling them to do more work at one time of the year and less at another. For example, parents can take more time off in the school holidays and GPs nearing retirement may wish to take longer holidays.

The scheme initially lasted for four years, providing GPs submitted their applications before 1 January 2004 and were in-post before 1 April 2004. It became three years for those applying thereafter. GPs submit an application form to NHS Professionals, which co-ordinates the administration of the scheme in England on behalf of the Department of Health. NHS Professionals then pass the application on to the relevant deanery.

The deanery determines eligibility of each applicant to join the scheme, and aims to be flexible to individual needs. Each GP will have a planned exit strategy from the start, which is agreed with an educational supervisor and the deanery. This is reviewed annually and GPs are expected to continue with a career in general practice after the scheme expires, unless they formally retire. Where possible, it is expected that employers of FCS GPs will make a commitment to their long-term employment once the GP has left the scheme. Where this is not possible the primary care trust (PCT) should work closely with local practices to identify appropriate alternatives. The deanery interviews all GPs entering the scheme, annually and when they leave the scheme.

Approval to employ an FCS GP

Both PCTs and practices can employ FCS GPs. Any practice, GMS or PMS, can be approved for employing an FCS GP providing it can demonstrate that it is working towards core criteria similar to the JCPTGP's minimum educational criteria for training practices, over an agreed time scale (*see* the modified Joint Committee criteria earlier in this chapter).

Each practice is individually matched to an FCS GP. Approval of a very experienced GP, for example a retired principal, will need a less rigorous practice assessment than for a relatively inexperienced GP who is working only a couple of sessions per week. Postgraduate training practices will automatically meet the criteria for hosting an FCS GP, but employment of an FCS GP will need to be sanctioned by the deanery in order to ensure that the educational component of the scheme is appropriate and generally to protect the needs of the FCS GP.

Deaneries must liaise closely with PCTs that employ FCS GPs to ensure that any placements are appropriate and that FCS GPs receive necessary support during their placement.

Educational aspects required of the FCS practice

- Adequate induction, educational input sufficient to meet the needs of the GP, named educational supervisor guiding the educational input, paid study leave for one session per week pro rata and weekly educational supervision.
- The practice must notify the deanery of any changes in premises, partnership or employment or educational arrangements of the FCS GP.
- If not a training practice, the practice Educational Facilitator undertakes preparation of the practice and themself for educating and employing an FCS GP.
- The educational input must be sufficient to meet the needs of the individual FCS GP and must be guided by a named educational facilitator.

Educational components of the scheme

- Each GP has a practice educational supervisor, whom the GP meets regularly in protected time.
- The practice can claim the full cost of eight sessions of education time (including on costs) for all FCS GPs, irrespective of the number of sessions that they work.
- Each GP will have an agreed PDP, which they will submit to the deanery on an annual basis along with their Appraisal Form 4 and their learning log.
- The FCS contract contains provision for one session of CPD for every eight clinical sessions worked, and this provision is in line with the new salaried GP's contract. The eight sessions of funded education is included within the time for CPD, but higher professional education (HPE) funding is in addition to this provision if the FCS GP is eligible.
- PDPs for FCS GPs should be locally agreed and depend upon the needs of individual GPs and their posts. The deanery gives some funding towards courses or books that are relevant to the PDP and it is suggested the FCS doctor approaches the practice or PCT for any additional funding.
- The practice is approved by the deanery

Other work that can be undertaken while on the scheme

GPs on the FCS are able to undertake additional work, such as educational or clinical assistant sessions, subject to the agreement of the deanery. The Department of Health has also opened the scheme to locums who wish to continue to undertake locum work while employed on the scheme. FCS GPs are able to undertake locum work in any capacity that is superannuable under the new contract. The expectation is that, where locum work is undertaken, the equivalent of four or five weekly FCS sessions are worked. Doctors who want to do fewer than four sessions on the FCS, but still do locum work, must discuss their individual circumstances with the deanery. The deanery exercises discretion and takes each GP's circumstances into account. This extends the reach of the FCS and provides locums with an employment route that enables them access to support for CPD, appraisal, revalidation and clinical governance arrangements.

Other benefits of the FCS

The scheme provides the FCS GP with £1050 towards professional expenses, such as defence organisation fees, and some doctors will attract a 'golden hello' payment. There is also a model contract, which provides terms and conditions no less beneficial than the new GMS salaried contract and reaches the improving working lives standards.

An employer committed to improving working lives:

- recognises the requirement for modern employment in practices
- understands that all staff work best for patients when they strike a healthy balance between work and other aspects of their life outside work
- develops a range of working arrangements that balance the needs of patients and services with the needs of staff
- values and supports staff
- provides personal and professional development and training opportunities that are accessible to all staff, irrespective of their working patterns
- provides a range of policies and practices that enable staff to manage a healthy balance between work and other commitments.

Benefits for the practice

Offering improved working conditions, through more family-friendly hours in an educationally supportive practice, is one of the strategies that a practice can use to attract and retain staff. The flexibility of the FCS can be used as a recruitment tool, enabling practices to be more creative about the way they work. GP partners who wish to reduce their commitment and work more flexibly as they near retirement can also use the scheme.

A percentage of the total employment costs are met by the Department of Health, on a sliding scale, depending on the length of time the FCS GP is in the scheme. The funds for this scheme come from a central source and do not therefore draw from other budgets available to practices and PCTs.

Comparison of the GP Retainer Scheme with the Flexible Career Scheme

Both schemes provide GPs with an opportunity to work in mainstream general practice while balancing their work and personal commitments. However, there are significant differences in both the aims of the schemes and in their detail.

The GP Retainer Scheme is designed to ensure that doctors who can only undertake a small amount of paid professional work keep in touch with general practice, retain their skills and progress their careers, with a view to returning to a substantive NHS general practice post in the future. Retainees are re-approved annually and may usually stay on the scheme for five years. The scheme is not intended for those planning a career in academic medicine, portfolio work or other sectors of clinical practice, and retainees may not undertake locum work. On the other hand, the FCS GP is able to undertake additional work as well as their two to five sessions on the FCS, and can also continue to undertake locum work while employed on the scheme. The FCS GP enjoys job continuity, with a contract for three or four years and there is an expectation that employers of FCS GPs will make commitment to their long-term employment once the GP has left the scheme, which is not the case for retainees.

The GP Retainer Scheme doctor should have well-founded personal, domestic or other reasons for undertaking only limited paid employment, and is supernumerary in the practice. In contrast, FCS GPs can take on a full workload while working flexibly within their negotiated hours. This gives the practice an opportunity to include the FCS GP in all aspects of the work of the practice.

The retainee GP may only undertake a limited amount of non-GMS or PMS work, normally no more than two extra sessions per week, whereas FCS GPs may have other employment outside their FCS sessions. The scheme has therefore proved popular with academics, retired GPs, GPs with a special interest in other clinical areas and portfolio GPs. The FCS has also the added benefit of flexibility, which allows GPs to organise their hours around their family or other commitments. In contrast, GP retainees must work a minimum of one session per week throughout the year, unless on leave.

The FCS GP's practice agrees to improving working lives standards and the model FCS contract, which is designed to provide fair employment conditions with similar terms to hospital colleagues. It has a continuity of service clause, thus valuing and retaining these GPs in the workforce[17] and, in addition, the practice receives funding towards maternity locums via the PCT. In contrast the retainer scheme contract does not provide for such beneficial terms and conditions, although this may change in the future.

The retainee GP receives £310 towards professional expenses, whereas the FCS GP receives £1050 and may also receive a 'golden hello'. Both GPs attract lower medical defence costs due to their membership of the schemes.

The Department of Health has said that the GP retainer scheme will continue to operate and complement the FCS, so GPs will have the maximum flexibility in identifying a scheme that best meets their individual needs.

Conclusion

These part-time educational schemes are essential to maintain the flexibility needed to retain the workforce in jobs that have traditionally embraced long hours and a 'macho' working culture, leading to much undisclosed ill-health, family disharmony, addiction and loss of doctors. We may be the first profession to have made this option available, and others, including law and practice nurses, may follow our lead.

The GP Retainer Scheme and the Flexible Career Scheme are producing a sub-group of doctors working in primary care, but this is not necessarily wrong if the users are happy and the scheme increases the retention of GPs in the current and future workforce. However, various studies[2,4,5,18] suggest that women continue to work part-time in general practice even when their domestic commitments diminish, which has implications for workforce planning.

References

1   Bradley H (1989) *Men's Work, Women's Work*. Polity Press, Cambridge.

2   Harvey J, Davison H, Winsland J *et al.* (1998) *Don't Waste Doctors: a report on wastage, recruitment and retention of doctors in the north west*. NHS Executive, Manchester.

3   NHS Executive (2000) *A Health Service of All the Talents: developing the NHS workforce*. Department of Health, London.

4   Allen I (1998) *Doctors and their Careers*. Policy Studies Institute, London.

5   Lambert TW and Goldacre JM (1998) Career destinations seven years on among doctors who qualified in the United Kingdom in 1988: postal questionnaire survey. *BMJ*. **317**: 1429–31.

6   Secretary of State for Health (1997) *The New NHS: modern and dependable*. The Stationary Office, London.

7   NHS Executive (1998) *GP Retainer Scheme*. Health Service Circular 1998/101. Department of Health, London.

8   Department of Health (2002) *GP Returners and Flexible Career Scheme for GPs*. Department of Health, London.

9   Department of Health and Social Security (1974) *Doctors' Retainer Scheme* Circular PM (79) 3. Department of Health and Social Security, London.

10 Department of Health (1991) *Women Doctors and their Careers: report of the Joint Working Party*. Department of Health, London.

11 Joint Committee on Postgraduate Training for General Practice (2004) *A Guide to Certification*. JCTGP, London.

12 Hastie A (2002) Assessment of the GP Retainer Scheme. *Education for Primary Care.* **13**: 233–8.

13 NHS Executive (2002) *NHS Professionals: flexible organisations, flexible staff.* HSC 2001/02. NHS Executive, Leeds.

14 Department of Health (2001) *Improving Working Lives Standard.* Department of Health, London.

15 Employment legislation (2002) *Flexible working – the right to request* (PL516 Rev 1) 6 April 2003.

16 NHS Executive (2000) *Flexible retirement.* HSC 2000/022. NHS Executive, Leeds.

17 Valuing doctors (2003) *NHS Magazine.* April: 22–3.

18 Davidson JM, Lambert TW and Goldacre MJ (1998) Career pathways and destinations 18 years on among doctors who qualified in the United Kingdom in 1977: postal questionnaire survey. *BMJ.* **31**: 1425–8.

CHAPTER 15

Managing the trainee doctor in difficulty

Elisabeth Paice and Victor Orton

Introduction

The emphasis in the National Health Service (NHS) is increasingly on delivering a safe, high-quality service to patients. Central to this changing culture is improving the way we deal with illness, misconduct or poor performance in healthcare workers. In all professions it is recognised that on occasion trainees may encounter difficulties. These may be manifested as ill health, misconduct, poor performance or dropping out of the system. The cost of training doctors is high and retention of doctors is therefore important to the service, but it cannot be at the expense of patient safety. Deaneries are responsible for the postgraduate training of doctors and dentists, and expect to be informed when problems arise, and if necessary to provide appropriate advice, educational support or referral. However, dealing with trainees in difficulty requires co-operation and a shared understanding among all those concerned and most of the detection, investigation, support and remediation will take place within trusts. In this chapter are discussed the contractual and legal context in which training occurs, the educational framework that supports training, some early signs that a trainee is at risk, the first steps that should be taken to investigate and deal with the concerns, the roles and responsibilities of the different individuals and organisations involved, and interventions that may prove helpful.

Contractual and legal framework

A doctor in training is usually employed by an NHS trust, and is subject to individual trust policies and procedures. The deanery has responsibility for managing the delivery of training across a programme, while the employer has responsibility for ensuring that employment matters, including disciplinary and performance issues, are dealt with appropriately. Each trainee has a continuing relationship with the deanery for the duration of the training programme. This relationship is separate from the contractual relationship with the trusts as employers.

Speciality Training Committees (STCs) are deanery committees where consultants representing the relevant royal college or faculty, consultants with training responsibilities in trusts and the deanery meet. STCs organise the specialist training programmes, and the recruitment and annual review of trainees. They act on behalf of the deanery and their decisions must be taken in accordance with national and deanery policies.[1]

Doctors employed in the training grades are issued with contracts of employment by trusts. In some deaneries there is one lead trust employing all doctors in training; in others, each trust is a separate employer. Trainees on rotational programmes have protection, under the Employment Rights Act 1996, of their continuity of service for statutory purposes, that is, unfair dismissal and redundancy rights, to be preserved for the duration of the training programme across all NHS employers. In addition, they are covered by the Human Rights Act, the Sex Discrimination Act, the Race Relations Act, the Disability Discrimination Act and European legislation, as well as Data Protection provisions. Recent and proposed changes in discrimination law have highlighted the responsibility of both employers and deaneries for ensuring that those in the position to provide or facilitate the provision of vocational training do so fairly, irrespective of disability, race, ethnicity, gender, sexual orientation, belief or age.

The assessment of trainees is undertaken by the educational supervisors and consultant trainers at the employing trust. In a number of specialities the royal colleges and their faculties have laid down criteria for assessment at the different levels of training. It is the responsibility of the employer to ensure that all its employees are treated fairly in accordance with trust policies and employment rights. The progress of trainees will be dependent on the outcome of the assessments provided at each placement, and the trainee may suffer serious detriment if these are not conducted fairly.

Each employer will have disciplinary procedures covering personal conduct issues and will follow HSC 2003/012[2] for professional competence and conduct issues. These procedures should not be used for dealing with poor performance issues, which can be handled through education and training. When there are health or conduct issues that call a doctor's fitness to practice into question, the trainee should be referred to the General Medical Council (GMC). Referral to the GMC for issues of poor performance alone would normally be appropriate only after all the available educational pathways have been exhausted.

The educational framework

Prevention is better than cure, and ensuring that a sound educational framework is in place wherever doctors are being trained is the first and most important step in any strategy to deal with trainees in difficulty.[3] Explicit educational quality standards should be included in the educational contract between the postgraduate dean and the trusts providing training. All trainees are entitled to regular appraisal, assessment and review of progress at each stage of their training. When such a framework is in place, it should be possible to deal locally with many issues of health, conduct, competence or performance (Box 15.1).

Box 15.1: The educational framework

- Induction, including speciality-specific induction
- Supervision, with an identified educational supervisor for each trainee
- Educational objective-setting within a short period of taking up the post;
- Personal development plans agreed between the trainee and the educational supervisor
- Regular appraisal with the supervising consultant
- Assessment of performance based on objective criteria and handled in a transparent manner
- Responsibility tailored to a realistic assessment of the trainee's experience and competence
- Pastoral support and confidential counselling services
- Mentoring by a supportive senior colleague if required or requested
- Occupational health services
- Remedial training opportunities when necessary
- Direct access to the postgraduate dean if required or requested

---

Early signs of the doctor in difficulty

On occasion it has taken a serious critical incident to highlight the fact that a trainee's behaviour or performance has been below standard for some time, whether because of stress, ill-health, substance abuse or poor professional skills, knowledge or attitudes.[4] Those responsible for the supervision of trainee doctors need to be alert to early signs of difficulty, so that action can be taken before patient care is put at risk.[5] To that end we report here the types of behaviours that in our experience have presaged serious problems, and merit concern.[6]

Unexplained absences

Arriving for work late, leaving early, not answering bleeps and excessive poorly explained sick leave are common features of doctors who are running into trouble. There may be many reasons for this behaviour, including: the early morning effects of depression or hangover; attempts to sort out complicated financial or relationship problems while at work; loss of confidence in making clinical decisions; or being at the receiving end of bullying or harassment. What we have learnt is that simply attempting to tackle punctuality, or failure to answer bleeps, is too superficial an approach. Trainees exhibiting this behaviour may have a serious underlying problem that needs to be explored possibly in parallel with appropriate disciplinary action.

Rigidity

Another early feature of the trainee in difficulty is rigidity. The doctor concerned may have difficulty dealing with uncertainty or ambiguity, an unwillingness to compromise in the face of competing priorities and intolerance of compromise in others. One consequence of rigidity is a slow work-rate that does not accelerate under pressure. This tends to infuriate colleagues, who feel forced to work faster and cut more corners themselves as a result. Another consequence is the writing of numerous letters of complaint to the management about the failures of others, out of proportion to the significance of the incidents. Features of trainees exhibiting rigidity include self-righteousness, rejection of any criticism and tendency to blame others.

Outbursts

Irritability is a common feature of stress, whatever the cause. Occasionally, the first indication of trouble has been an uncontrollable outburst of anger in a clinical setting – what might be called 'ward rage'. These may include flare-ups with medical colleagues, nurses or patients. Sometimes the trigger for the outburst is some real or imagined criticism or slight.

Failure to gain the trust of others

When a trainee's competence or reliability is below the expected standard, colleagues or patients may recognise a problem before it comes to the attention of the consultant. Patients may ask to see a different doctor, nursing staff may go over the head of the individual to ask the opinion of more senior colleagues, and peers may attempt to avoid being on duty with the doctor concerned. Supervising consultants should also be alert to the possibility of bullying or harassment when certain trainees are marginalised by colleagues. Whatever the reason, being bypassed or marginalised at work is isolating and saps confidence. Serious attention should be paid if it is discovered that this is happening, and action should be taken to ensure either that the trainee is enabled to play a full part in the team, or that deficiencies are addressed.

Problems of probity

Probity is one of the duties of a doctor, and the sort of casual 'economy with the truth' that might be tolerated in another walk of life should ring alarm bells in a doctor in training. An example is in writing a curriculum vitae, where exaggeration of competence or previous experience might be the norm in some careers, but could endanger patient safety if it secured the doctor a post beyond his or her capabilities. Trivial, casual or minor degrees of dishonesty should not be overlooked, as they may lead to more serious breaches.

Lack of insight

It is a common finding that trainees whose behaviour or performance is giving rise to concern may be unaware of the problem, and they may deny any short-comings which are brought to their attention, often counter-challenging with allegations of discrimination, bullying or substandard training. This makes dealing with the issues more difficult, and may lead to reluctance on the part of those in a supervisory capacity to tackle problems at an early stage. There is evidence to suggest that insight does not come from feedback, however forceful or consistent, but from education and training about the correct way to perform or behave.[7] Absence of insight should not be seen as a personality trait, but as a learning need, and handled accordingly.[8]

Poor clinical performance

Poor clinical performance in trainees is usually considered an educational issue and handled locally by intensified training and supervision. Trainees are, after all, there to learn. It is only when performance consistently falls well below the standard expected, or when a trainee refuses to accept criticism or to make efforts to improve, that the deanery becomes involved. The sorts of performance issues that come up most frequently include: poor note-keeping or prescription writing; failure to follow protocols; inappropriate investigations; failure to recognise or respond to the urgency of a clinical situation; and problems with practical procedures. The steps in dealing with poor performance in the workplace are set out in Box 15.2.

Box 15.2: First steps in managing poor performance

- Address unsatisfactory performance at the time it occurs, bringing it to the attention of the trainee and asking for an explanation; do not wait for the next appraisal
- Be clear about the ways in which the behaviour or performance observed differs from that expected of the trainee; have examples
- Explore with the trainee the cause of the problem, including any personal or professional pressures, and offer support and referral to occupational health where appropriate
- Interview in private and keep all discussions confidential; offer the trainee the opportunity to include a third party for support
- Agree a plan for improvement with a reasonable timeframe (e.g. three or six months)
- Provide supervision, training, development or support to assist the trainee to improve
- Introduce regular review sessions (e.g. fortnightly or monthly), with clear objectives or targets to be achieved
- Make it clear to the trainee why this heightened level of supervision is necessary, and how long it is expected to last
- Document the process, all discussions, expectations and outcomes; share with the trainee what has been written
- If after review, performance has not improved, consider other avenues, such as change of training environment; targeted or remedial training, or disciplinary action, depending on the nature of the problem
- Human resources and occupational health professionals will be a source of useful support and advice and should be consulted

---

Targeted and remedial training

Targeted training

When targeted training is deemed necessary, this fact should be recorded (use RITA Form D)[9] with a start date and an expected review date, and the objectives to be met within that timescale. Objectives should be set that can be justified by reference to the curriculum for the training programme being undertaken, or to the GMC document, *Good Medical Practice*. Where possible, targeted training should be provided within the training post or rotation to which the trainee had been assigned, in order to avoid disruption within the programme. If this is not possible, because the educational opportunities or the appropriate level of supervision are not available, it may be necessary to move a trainee to a different post or trust. Such a move should be taken in consultation with the trainee, the educational supervisors and the employing trusts concerned. The potential impact on the training of other trainees should be taken into account. The receiving educational supervisor and human resources director should be informed in writing of the proposed arrangements and be given written information about the areas of practice that give rise to concern. This information may be necessary to protect patient safety, and it is certainly necessary to ensure optimum educational supervision. The trainee should be advised that this will happen and should receive a copy of the information.

Remedial training

Remedial training may be required where performance has been so far below the standard expected that repeat or exceptional training is necessary and progress must be delayed while this is provided. Such decisions should not be taken lightly, or without robust objective evidence of unsatisfactory progress. The trainee should be offered the opportunity to discuss this evidence, and to submit any evidence to support a contrary view. The decision to extend training and provide remediation should be taken in consultation with the deanery and based on evidence from more than one supervisor.[10] The decision, the reasons for it, and the evidence taken into account should be well-documented (*see* RITA Form E).[9] As above, the timescale for review, and the objectives to be met within that timescale should be agreed and documented. An appeal process for specialist registrars (SpRs) is set out in the *Guide to Specialist Registrar Training*.[9] A similar process should be followed where the need for remedial training is appealed against in more junior grades. All trusts, as partners within the NHS, will be expected to accept their fair share of responsibility for accepting trainees with difficulties.

Withdrawal from training

The training of doctors represents a considerable investment of public money and every effort should be made to help doctors in difficulty, as long as this is consistent with patient safety and high-quality care. Very occasionally, the postgraduate dean, acting on evidence submitted, and in consultation with the trainers, will determine that a doctor is no longer suitable to remain in a training programme. Under those circumstances, the trainee will be withdrawn from the programme and the contract of employment ended.

Disciplinary procedures

The deanery must be informed in writing by the trust of any disciplinary action being taken against a trainee. Assurances will be sought on the following:

- that the trust is following an agreed disciplinary procedure that conforms to best practice and is legally sustainable
- that the trainee has been advised on representation
- that national guidelines are followed where a trainee is excluded
- that pastoral support and guidance is being offered.

The deanery will not normally be involved on disciplinary or appeal panels in any disciplinary procedures taken by a trust against a trainee. The deanery, or the royal college or faculty, may provide advice and information on issues relating directly to training or education. Depending on the outcome of any disciplinary action, the postgraduate dean may advise the trust of any training or educational needs relevant to the particular case.[11]

On occasions it may be necessary for the trust or deanery to advise the GMC of substantiated allegations against a trainee. In such situations the trainee must be advised of such action. If the doctor leaves the employment of the trust, with serious concerns about his or her performance still unresolved, the medical director may wish to contact the regional director of public health, who may in turn issue an 'Alert Letter' (HSG (97) 36), which will cascade out to all trusts. This will state that anyone considering employing the individual should contact the medical director originating the alert. The doctor should be advised in writing by recorded delivery that this action is being taken.

Serious untoward incidents involving a doctor in training

On occasion a trainee may make an isolated but serious medical mistake. Such situations can be highly stressful for all involved and may lead to a formal inquiry or even manslaughter charges. The trainee concerned is likely to be distraught by the event, and urgent consideration should be given to removing him or her from clinical responsibilities and offering psychological support. The trainee should be advised to write down the events while fresh, but to seek legal advice before submitting a formal statement. A consultant mentor should be identified to offer the trainee advice and support. The outcome of any inquiry or disciplinary should be made known to the next employing trust and the deanery on a confidential basis, in the interests of patient safety and of appropriate educational supervision. Trainees should always be informed of any information being passed on about them.

Ill health, substance abuse and unprofessional behaviour

Health matters should be dealt with outside of the disciplinary procedures through the trust's occupational health processes. Where the doctor's fitness to practise is impaired by a physical or mental condition the GMC should be advised. The deanery will need to be informed in writing. Doctors found to be abusing drugs or alcohol, or behaving in a seriously unprofessional manner, should be referred to the GMC and, where appropriate, the 'Sick Doctors' scheme. The postgraduate dean should be informed in writing of any such action. It may be necessary for the police to be involved in appropriate circumstances, for example assault, theft, fraud or misrepresentation.

Transfer of information from trust to trust

Throughout a doctor's training each placement, from the first pre-registration house-officer (PRHO) post to the final SpR post, should be seen as part of the educational continuum. The ability to demonstrate competencies and conduct appropriate to the level of training forms part of this continuum. It is recognised that on occasion, where disciplinary action has been taken to address deficiencies in areas of performance or conduct, intensified supervision or targeted training may still be required when the trainee comes to the end of a placement. The educational supervisor at the next placement will need to be made aware of these ongoing special training needs.

It is essential that information about any disciplinary or performance issue and a written statement about the facts of the case, be transferred to the next employing trust. Reference should be made to any formal action taken against the trainee, detailing the nature of the incident triggering such action, the allegations that were upheld (but not those that were dismissed) and the outcome of the disciplinary along with any ongoing targeted or remedial training. Under these exceptional circumstances the information should be transferred, with the knowledge of the postgraduate dean and the doctor in training, to the human resources director of the next employing trust, who will inform the appropriate educational supervisor. This also applies to current non-expired disciplinary warnings, which will continue to carry weight in the receiving trust. If there has been no disciplinary procedure, but there are ongoing special educational or supervisory needs, the information may be best transferred via the postgraduate dean to the receiving clinical tutor or other educational lead.

The trainee has a right to know what information is being transferred and to be given an opportunity to challenge its accuracy but not to prevent the information being transferred. The trainee should meet with the educational supervisor at the next trust early on in the placement to discuss objectives and agree a timetable of progress. Regular appraisals should take place and a formal review of progress and performance should be undertaken at the end of the first three months in the new post and a report sent to the postgraduate dean and copied to the trainee. The trainee has a right to know whether performance is now considered adequate or not and the postgraduate dean needs to consider whether the trainee has the ability to progress through the programme.

Support for trainees in difficulty

Trainees joining a training programme should be offered information about the pastoral and psychological support available to them, at trust, deanery and national level. Such information is often included in induction packs, but rarely remembered by trainees. The information should therefore be made available also on notice boards in education centres and other accessible places. Clinical tutors and educational supervisors should also be aware of the availability of support. The trust's occupational health service will be very experienced in dealing with psychological stress as well as other health issues, and should be consulted when trainees begin to run into difficulty. Confidential counselling services outside the trust are provided in many deaneries, for example the MedNet service in London, which takes self-referrals from both trainees and trainers in need of psychological support.

Trainees who have complaints about their training, or about perceived discrimination, bullying or harassment, should normally use internal trust procedures to raise these. The clinical tutor is the appropriate person within the trust with whom to raise concerns about training. Alternatively, the speciality training programme director or STC chair may be appropriate for an SpR.

There will be occasions when trainees feel that local trust or speciality-based procedures have not dealt with their concerns adequately, or where they are reluctant to raise them for fear of retribution. Under those circumstances, the postgraduate dean will always be prepared to arrange a confidential meeting and to advise and support the trainee through the appropriate procedures to deal with the problems raised.

Conclusion

Managing trainee doctors who have become ill, disillusioned or dysfunctional, and whose careers have derailed as a consequence, is a difficult and usually unrewarding business. As with patient care, prevention is better than cure. Where prevention is not possible, early diagnosis and intervention leads to better results than late diagnosis and heroic treatment. Much of our experience in the deanery has necessarily been with trainees whose behaviour has caused serious concern. In most of these cases there was earlier evidence that trouble was brewing, which went unrecognised, unchallenged and undocumented. The deanery has put considerable effort into working with consultant trainers to raise awareness of these early signs. Evidence is beginning to accumulate that in a proportion of cases early recognition and support can be effective in getting careers back on track. Where the outcome has not been positive, at least early recognition, discussion and documentation of problems has helped in reaching a robust outcome that has withstood challenge.

References

1   Committee of Postgraduate Medical Deans (2000) *A Guide to the Management and Quality Assurance of Postgraduate Medical and Dental Education.* COPMED, London. (www.copmed. org.uk/Publications/GreenGuide)

2   Department of Health (2004) *Maintaining High Professional Standards in the Modern NHS: a framework for the initial handling of concerns about doctors and dentists in the NHS.* HSC 2003/ 012. Department of Health, London. (www.dh.gov.uk/PublicationsAndStatistics/ LettersAndCirculars/HealthServiceCirculars)

3   Moss F and Paice E (1999) Getting things right for the doctor in training. In: Firth-Cozens J and Payne R (eds) *Stress in Health Professionals.* John Wiley & Sons, Chichester.

4   Yao DC and Wright SM (2001) The challenge of problem residents. *Journal of General Internal Medicine.* **16**: 486–92.

5   Paice E (2000) Early identification, diagnosis and response. In: Ghodes E, Mann S and Johnson P (eds) *Doctors and Their Health: who heals the healers?* Reed Healthcare, Surrey.

6   Paice E and Orton V (2004) Early signs of the trainee in difficulty. *Hospital Medicine.* **65**: 238–40

7   Kruger J and Dunning D (1999) Unskilled and unaware of it: how difficulties in recognising one's own incompetence lead to inflated self-assessments. *Journal of Personality and Social Psychology.* **77**: 1121–34.

8   Hays RB, Jolly BC, Caldon LJM *et al.* (2002) Is insight important? Measuring capacity to change performance. *Medical Education.* **36**: 965–71.

9   Department of Health (1998) *A Guide to Specialist Registrar Training.* Department of Health, London.

10 Sim F (1999) Record of In-Training assessment (RITA): a look at ethical issues in assessment. *Hospital Medicine.* **60**: 676–8.

11 Paice E, Orton V and Appleyard J (1999) Managing trainee doctors in difficulty. *Hospital Medicine.* **60**: 130–3.

CHAPTER 16

Deanery performance work in primary care

Julia Whiteman and Alex Trompetas

Introduction

Deaneries have an important role to play in supporting general practitioners (GPs) whose performance has been identified as being below that which is required to provide an acceptable standard of service delivery in primary care. In addition, deaneries have a responsibility to work constructively and in co-operation with the other organisations involved, including primary care trusts (PCTs), the National Clinical Assessment Authority (NCAA)[1] and the General Medical Council (GMC).[2] The work involved requires consistency within a framework of equal opportunity and sensitivity to the emotional welfare of the poorly performing GP who may well have found the assessment procedures leading to the identification of poor performance quite bruising. In addition, accuracy is required with information-gathering and recording, and integrity whereby the tension is held between the situation presented and information which is shared with other professionals and agencies. All this must be maintained while frequently working in a variety of perverse situations – poorly performing GPs often work as part of a poorly performing multiprofessional team and in deprived socio-economic areas where under investment, large list sizes and difficulty recruiting and retaining practice staff has become an all too familiar picture. Equally, poor performance can often lie alongside health and conduct issues that can compromise any educational input prescribed to address the areas of concern.

In this chapter deanery involvement in GP underperformance at a local level is considered, as part of its continuing professional development (CPD) work and centrally through the performance unit that responds to referrals from the GMC, NCAA and PCTs, as well as self-referrals. In both aspects the roles and responsibilities of deanery educators are observed and a range of support and remedial intervention is suggested.

The contribution the deanery can make to support poor performers in general practice

GP deaneries are the organisations that provide education and training for the GP workforce, both locally in the PCTs and centrally through CPD initiatives, both clinically and educationally based. Hence, it is important that they be involved in all cases of underperformance where there is the possibility that educational needs exist which will otherwise bar progress towards appropriate performance standards. Underperformance caused by pure educational need rarely exists in isolation. The other GMC categories of conduct and health often run in parallel, and they can take precedence over educational needs if, for instance, the situation includes criminal activity in the case of conduct, or illness so that the GP is unable to learn even if willing to do so.

Local involvement in underperformance

The tutor network provides the link at local levels between the deanery, PCTs and GP CPD. Traditionally, tutors have been providers of continuing medical education (CME) for GPs, but latterly they have moved towards a more strategic involvement in educational provision for primary care at PCT level. GP appraisal has shaped the direction and thrust of their work, with tutors acting as advisers to appraisers and appraisees on personal development plans (PDPs) and to the PCTs about meeting developmental needs identified as a result of the appraisal process.

Therefore, although it is inappropriate for tutors to be involved in the identification and assessment of poor performance, as it is outside their role and expertise, it is entirely appropriate to involve local tutors to help plan a remedial course of action once poor performance has been identified. With the consent and full engagement of the GP concerned, a tutor could help draw up a PDP appropriate for the situation presented, which is realistic and achievable within the timescales set. The tutor might also help the GP to identify a mentor to support them further in their endeavours.

PCTs have their local groups set up to identify, assess and manage underperformance. Assessment of underperformance will result in an action plan, ranging from no action to referral to the GMC with an educational prescription for remedial measures occurring in between. The NCAA has provided guidelines for local performance processes.

Central deanery performance support unit

The deanery performance support unit (PSU) can become involved in a case of underperformance, either through a direct referral from an organisation such as a PCT, NCAA or the GMC, as a self-referral, or as a request for advice from another deanery colleague working in the locality.

Referrals coming from the GMC are likely to have a long and complicated history, which may have had a damaging and demoralising effect on the GP concerned. The deanery will therefore be expected to provide educational input to someone who may well have become disenfranchised from primary care and from GP colleagues. It is much simpler and more rewarding to be drawn early on, when the GP is still in practice, or has only recently been removed, and where he or she has local contacts who can provide opportunities for work-based support and learning in a familiar environment.

When advice is sought from the PSU it is often done on the basis that the GP concerned remains anonymous. This is rightly so, as poor performance might not have been proven and indeed might not exist; the risks of labelling a GP inappropriately have potentially damaging and libellous consequences. However, the deanery has a duty to support colleagues working in primary care and needs to have the facility to provide high-quality advice on local remedial actions and educational procedures. Undoubtedly, having good working relationships and trust with colleagues is essential for advice and prompt referrals, and such relationships should be nurtured through whatever means are appropriate. In London, where there are five strategic health authority sectors, the three members of the PSU accepting referrals unit have their work divided on a sector basis to help develop local knowledge and contacts to a greater level.

Context for this work

Work with GP underperformance cannot take place in isolation. The deanery is part of an important network that includes the following.

- The GMC, with its statutory responsibility to regulate the medical profession and ensure that the standards of *Good Medical Practice*[4] are upheld.
- The NCAA.
- PCTs, as organisations responsible for managing GP performer lists and with the power invested in them through the Health and Social Care Act, have been able to – and have had to be seen to – act more swiftly where there is the suggestion of GP underperformance.
- Workforce Development Confederations (WDCs), with their responsibility for maintaining and developing the primary care workforce through periods of low recruitment when a poor performer is lost from the workforce, can leave 2000 or so patients without a GP.
- The general public since, at the time of writing, week by week the impact of the Shipman inquiry and other high-profile media cases has led to public demand for greater professional accountability.[5]

When reviewing its role in performance work, the deanery must take into account recent changes in primary care development and accountability, principally the debate about GP appraisal and revalidation, and the emergence of the PDP as a more meaningful route towards professional development. Increased accountability through clinical governance work, and PCT-held GP performer lists may increase demands on remedial education in order to keep GPs working. This may be particularly relevant for GPs who had been working as GP non-principals as they were outside the postgraduate education allowance system and initially not included in GP appraisal

What can the deanery offer an underperforming GP?

Whether working as part of the PSU or locally the deanery can offer an underperformer a range of resources. These include the following.

Realistic advice

By the time someone is in contact with the deanery, either through self-referral or referral from another organisation, he or she will have had to face facts about their performance level. Whether or not the situation is acknowledged and the steps needed to remediate matters are appreciated it will have been a difficult process for the GP concerned. They may well have lost professional status and standing, and this, as with any other bereavement process, will result in a series of reactions: denial, anger and depression, before acceptance can allow the GP to move forward. Compounding this, in the case of GMC referrals, will be the sanctions meted out and a timeframe to work to. Are the goals achievable and is the effort needed realistic in the context of their overall plans *vis-à-vis* retirement or other life events? Have they the financial resources to meet their needs and are there other barriers to their progress? As with Maslow's hierarchy of need[6] individuals need to feel that they have love, belonging and at least some measure of esteem before they achieve self-actualisation and move forward. Denial of the situation they are in will waste time and resources, and will further marginalise them from the mainstream. Hence a supportive approach with a thorough and honest appraisal of the true situation from a neutral perspective is necessary and probably something best offered by the PSU.

Personal development planning

There are many examples and templates for PDPs. The essence of a PDP is to address educational needs that have been identified, acknowledged and prioritised in a way that is meaningful to the individual concerned so that he or she is able to bring about a positive change in their knowledge base or skills, and are able to achieve a higher level of competency in their work. The PDP must be relevant to the educational needs of the individual GP, meaningful for their future professional intentions, realistic and achievable.

The individual GP's performance analysis should be completed prior to their referral to the deanery and this would be used as part of their educational needs analysis. However, other than in the situation of a self-referral, a performance assessment resulting in a statement of educational needs is likely to have been conducted by a third party and the findings may or may not be acknowledged by the GP concerned. Whilst at risk of labouring this point, it cannot be emphasised too strongly that if the GP is unwilling to address the needs, or cannot understand their basis, it is unrealistic to expect them to be able to address the needs and hence including these needs in a PDP at this point is illogical. Learning needs analysis, negotiation around personal circumstances and a commitment to address them are the critical stages of personal development planning. Once the PDP is agreed the PSU will need to offer support to the GP in whatever context they have for their work. It may well include attendance at a 'Fresh Start' course as described below. Either way helping to identify local support through mentorship and supervision will enhance learning, in particular the transfer of learning into practice, and therefore quality of service delivery (Figure 16.1).

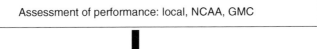

Assessment of performance: local, NCAA, GMC

- Individual remedial training, preferably near or at place of work
- Fresh start modality, i.e. clinical or personal management or organising the practice, according to areas initially identified by assessment
- Creation of education plan, with specific training and education goals to achieve

- Connecting with education network
- Sharing of education needs analysis and education plan
- Working on training needs using local and deanery input
- Review of training and education progress after set periods of time, i.e. six months or one year

Figure 16.1 Assessment, education needs and the development of a personal development plan (PDP).

Lastly, the PDP provides a means of monitoring progress against the agreed aims and objectives, and it therefore provides a framework for reporting back to referring bodies on the progress made by the GP concerned.

Link with GP appraisal

At the time of writing, GP appraisal is a formative tool designed to help GPs review their work in context and, through the construction of a PDP, move forward in a way that is relevant to them and the needs of their practice.[7] GP underperformers are entitled to the same educationally sound developmental appraisal process and, through the support offered by the deanery, should be able to participate in this process in a way that offers the opportunity of supported reflection in a non-judgemental setting.

Fresh start

The London Deanery has developed a flexible modular course called 'Fresh Start' as a programme to address the needs of GPs with difficulties. The initial Fresh Start programme was a full-time, week-long course at a venue selected so as to be slightly secluded and with facilities for the attendees to stay overnight. Great emphasis was placed on teamworking and forming effective groups through working together in the different modules. GPs with a mixture of problems, including conduct and health issues, have applied to attend, and such variety of cases generated the need for vigorous screening of applicants often by a mini-interview and a careful consideration of their circumstances to establish whether they would benefit from attending the programme.

The main areas of expertise and development within the course were:

- simulated surgery
- communication or consultation skills
- dilemmas, including ethics and the law
- practice organisation.

The above areas of concern were the result of anecdotal evidence from referrals to the PSU.

Although a six-monthly, weekly standard course provided time to cover a wide range of curriculum topics in a tried and trusted format, there was not the time nor flexibility to link educational provision to learning need. Hence the course has developed into a series of two-day modules in each of the main areas as described above. These modules are run at different times through the year and in different locations around London. This allows more focused learning and more time spent on each module. It may also be possible to establish more concrete outcomes by addressing smaller groups and linking more closely with PCTs and performance advisory groups in different areas.

Discussions with partner organisations, including the NCAA, the GMC, London local medical committees (LMCs) and National Association of Primary Care Educators (NAPCE) have helped to further develop and define the content of these modules, which include the following.

- Clinical skills, including medical records, consultation and communicating with the patient, clinical knowledge, clinical decision-making and ability to function during surgery faced with a variety of clinical problems.
- Practice administration and organisational skills. This looks at some of the individual organisational skills and also focuses on systems such as practice organisation and utilisation of the primary healthcare team.
- Ethics and the law. This module looks at the wider framework of the NHS, within which primary care functions. It includes input at individual level of ethical and legal considerations as consequence of clinical practice. It looks at some of the dilemmas and wider issues behind clinical decisions.

GPs attending the Fresh Start course have to agree to share the findings of the course with supervisors and the referring authority, and the course should be part of their PDP.

How can the deanery equip itself to deal with the challenges of GP underperformance?

The deanery needs clarity around the contribution it can make in providing remedial support with performance cases, and this needs to be clearly communicated across the organisation and with the other agencies, both locally and nationally, as described above. Such clarity should be negotiated to ensure it beds in well within the deanery's educational and developmental ethos, meets educational needs and is synchronous with the approaches of the other agencies.

Providing for the supporters

'Supporters' here is used as a broad term that includes all those who come up against the challenges of managing underperformance, either as a principal component of their work in the PSU, or as a tutor, course organiser or director finding underperformance as a consequence of their work. In order to perform to a satisfactory, fair and safe standard they need training and support themselves for their work.

The training needed can be broadly divided into:

- developing understanding of the legislation and statutory frameworks
- how to prepare reports using evidence gathered and present this in an acceptable form, either as a written report or in person at a hearing

- developing and refining educational skills to be effective at guiding a remedial GP in the different stages of personal development planning.

None of the above are specific skills for performance work and they would be part of the normal skills base of a tutor or deanery director. The knowledge base to understand the approach to managing cases can be developed experientially through casework and more didactic sources.

The challenge with performance work is found in the complexities of the problems confronted, in individuals who are often demotivated, lacking in insight and divorced from the process of reflective practice and learning. Therefore those involved in handling performance cases need space to reflect upon and discuss their work, to share problems and solutions. Cases being worked on provide rich learning material for discussion and reflection. There are huge benefits of regular case discussion meetings to build on understanding of performance issues, working relationships and trust.

Providing remedial support to struggling GPs is a challenging part of deanery business, but one that can make a meaningful contribution to retaining GPs who work to high standards in the workforce.

References

1 www.ncaa.nhs.uk

2 www.gmc-uk.org

3 National Clinical Assessment Authority (2002) *NCAA Handbook*. NCAA, London.

4 General Medical Council (2001) *Good Medical Practice*. GMC, London.

5 www.the-shipman-enquiry.org.uk

6 Maslow AH (1943) A theory of human motivation. *Psychological Review*. **50**: 370–96.

7 www.gpappraisal.nhs.uk

CHAPTER 17

Assessment

Nav Chana and Colin Stern

Driving imperatives

The public's opinion of the National Health Service (NHS) in general, and of the medical profession in particular, has fallen significantly in the last decade. The press has seized on scandals such as the Bristol paediatric cardiac surgery fiasco, Harold Shipman's murderous career, Rodney Ledward's cavalier treatment of his patients and the irresponsible retention of children's body parts at Alder Hey to create an image of an uncaring, poorly skilled and insensitive profession.[1,2,3,4]

At the same time, the profession has woken up to the need to modernise its approach to learning and develop ways in which the skills and attributes acquired by doctors in training can be more reliably guaranteed.[5,6] A great deal of work has been done to identify how best this may be achieved, and this chapter will bring together the most suitable tools and methods for assessing the progress made by doctors in training towards best performance.

Although the incidents that led to these improvements were dramatic, there are important imperatives for their introduction in everyday clinical practice. Central to better training and assessment is patient care, the core value of the London Deanery.[7] Better public perception of the health service is integral to patient care, because good reports spread more widely and efficiently by word of mouth than via the press. Regular reports of good practice and outcomes are important to politicians, although a single lapse often has a disproportionately adverse effect on them. Lastly, the profession is notoriously dissatisfied with the developing skills of those in training and this educational reform must convince them that the coming generation of doctors will be more reliably assessed as competent.

Principles of assessment

The Postgraduate Medical Education and Training Board (PMETB) is assuming responsibility for approving the education and training of doctors and will issue the Certificate of Completion of Training (CCT). The PMETB has established a sub-group on assessment, chaired by Dame Lesley Southgate, which has agreed principles and standards for assessment to which any system introduced for this purpose should conform.[8,9] The principles are as follows.

- The assessment system must be fit for a range of purposes.
- The content of the assessment (sample of knowledge, skills and attitudes) will be based on curricula for postgraduate training which themselves are referenced to all of the areas of good medical practice.
- The methods used within the programme will be selected in the light of the purpose and content of that component of the assessment framework.
- The methods used to set standards for classification of trainee's performance or competence must be transparent and in the public domain.
- Assessments must provide relevant feedback.
- Assessors or examiners will be recruited against criteria for performing the tasks they undertake.
- There will be lay input in the development of assessment.
- Documentation will be standardised and accessible nationally.

Each of these principles has been assigned a set of related standards that should be met. Assessments should take place using methods that have been shown to be valid, reliable, evidence-based and cost-effective. Skills and competencies relevant to the career should be tested and match progression through training, but be unique to each skill tested and without gaps. As experience with the methods grows following pilot studies, norm-referencing will be introduced, using standardised, national documentation.

The PMETB subgroup suggested a variety of ways in which assessments might be made in the workplace. One set is the systematic observation of clinical practice, such as by direct observation or by video. Another set requires the judgements of multiple assessors, including: consulting with simulated patients; case record review including outpatient letters; case-based discussions; oral presentations; 360° peer assessment; patient surveys; audit projects; and critical incident reviews.

Some of these methods tend to be employed in formal college examinations, for example consulting with standardised patients.[10] Others, such as audit projects and presentations, are routinely undertaken by doctors in training and lend themselves to formal methods of rating. A few, such as structured cased-based discussion and 360° appraisals, are especially relevant to the assessment of skills and competencies. In addition, the direct observation of clinical practice needs the use of a standardised method of assessment, such as the mini-clinical examination (Mini-CEX), which is similar to the traditional short case assessment.

The purpose of assessment

In recommending the above principles and standards for an assessment system for postgraduate medical training, the PMETB subgroup defines an assessment system as:

> An integrated set of assessments which is in place for the entire postgraduate training programme, and which supports the curriculum. It may comprise different methods, and be implemented either as national examinations, or as assessments in the workplace. The balance between these two approaches principally relates to the relationship between competence and performance. Competence (can do) is necessary but not sufficient for performance (does do), and as experience increases so performance based assessment becomes more important.[8]

The relevance of any assessment used should be achieved by an explicit link to the curriculum. In the past, the curriculum has been interpreted narrowly as meaning a specified course of study or a written syllabus. Today, the definition is much wider and includes all the planned learning experiences of a school or educational institution.[10] The curriculum should focus upon outcomes,[11] and outcomes should be expressed in terms of the demonstration of appropriate clinical behaviours, rather than divorced from the development of skills.[12] This leads to the notion of developing competency statements, which can then be tested by a planned system of assessment.

The need for competency-based assessment has been highlighted by the Chief Medical Officer (CMO) and provides a political driver for change as well as an educational one.[13] The CMO also highlights the importance of royal college examinations in the continuum of training and their place as part of the educational process. However, the assessment of competence must be distinguished from the assessment of performance: both are key qualities, although the latter permits the comparison of the better performer with the average one in a workplace setting.

Miller's pyramid provides clear challenges when assessing clinical competence and performance.[14] Wilkinson *et al.*[15] suggested that the aim of assessment of doctors in training should be to measure their performance in a valid and reliable way.

When attempting to gain a global view of a practitioner's performance it is likely that a variety of methods will be required. Southgate *et al.*[16] propose a selection of assessments based on patient-based data, peer review, clinical outcomes, performance testing (ensuring that competence exists beyond five to 10 indicator conditions) and self-assessment.

Emphasis is placed on ensuring that a range of measures and indicators contribute to a 'broad performance profile' of individual doctors, which reflects the actual workload of clinicians within their working environments and that 'indicator decisions are selected according to evidence that decisions have critical impacts on outcomes'.

Workplace-based assessments seem likely to be shown to be valid, chiefly through the high authenticity of testing doctors in the environment in which they work, but questions have been raised about the reliability of these methods. For example, when attempting to measure the highest level of the pyramid using workplace-based methods the 'sensible' assumption that 'assessments of actual practice are a much better reflection of routine performance than assessments done under test conditions' remains 'unproven'.[17]

The great difficulty of attempting to measure 'actual performance' in a reliable way has led to the use of simulated encounters, including the use of standardised patients in high stakes tests[18] and as incognito attenders.[10,19] The validity of 360° appraisals in measuring performance has also been demonstrated.[20]

It is apparent that there remains considerable debate over the merits of performance testing, either by using work-based methods or by simulated encounter. Furthermore, in the context of a high stakes assessment (i.e. where an inappropriate pass represents the greatest risk to the stakeholders) it would seem logical to consider the development of a variety of assessment methods, which are complementary and part of a global assessment framework.

Defining what should be tested

In addition to identifying how doctors in training may be assessed, we need to think about what qualities should be assessed. The standard criteria to be used are those enshrined in *Good Medical Practice*,[9] in which the General Medical Council (GMC) identified the professional virtues that all doctors must demonstrate and they have become central to appraisal, assessment, validation and revalidation. The themes include: good professional practice and continuous professional development (CPD); good relationships with patients and colleagues; teaching, training and research; probity and health. Taking them as a basis for assessment, specific areas of competence which are amenable to performance testing using an evidence-based approach may be identified..

Communication

Effective communication is central to good clinical practice. The ability to unravel the clinical basis of a patient's problem depends upon effective, active listening.[21] Describing the cause of the trouble and recommending a course of treatment requires doctors to understand how patients see themselves and to use language that matches their circumstances. At the same time, doctors must be able to listen to and to inform the other members of the team effectively.

Clinical skills

New styles of undergraduate curricula concentrate on self-directed learning and communication skills.[22] The acquisition of basic clinical skills remains important, but the time available to learn them has been compressed. Consequently, the early years of clinical practice have become more crucial in developing the skills of clinical examination and those of diagnosis and management. These attributes must be evaluated, most especially during foundation programmes.[23]

Technical skills

Some technical skills are integral to clinical diagnosis and management, such as venepuncture, intravenous cannulation and the insertion of long intravenous lines, chest drainage and lumbar puncture. The most appropriate assessors of these competences are usually nursing staff or middle grade medical staff. The craft specialities of medicine, such as cardiology and the many varieties of surgery, require skills that doctors must acquire in order to practise effectively. Consultants, most often educational supervisors, best evaluate these skills.

Learning

In the past formal education has too often been the only criterion of learning. Doctors in training need to attend courses to learn specific aspects of their chosen field, and their records of attendance presently attest to this need. It would be more valuable to develop ways to evaluate improvements in practice, which flow from formal learning, and methods of achieving this are available. Research has been held in similar esteem, and often for its own sake, but we are moving into an era where more direct evaluations of the beneficial effects of research upon clinical practice are becoming important.

Professional performance

Trained doctors must have skills other than the clinical and technical in order to practise their chosen speciality. They will work in teams, undertake management and teaching responsibilities, give lectures, take part in audit and risk management and assume a variety of other roles. These skills have not been a conventional part of the education of doctors, but the London Deanery has developed a modular course, 'Managing Life', which is designed to impart them. An important element in this course is that it is delivered to participants from a variety of healthcare professions. The multidisciplinary nature of the course is crucial in developing the teamworking skills that modern doctors need.

Medical education is like a relay race and every skilled practitioner should be engaged continuously in passing his or her skills on to succeeding generations. We have become aware that this requires skill in teaching, and have begun to formulate the teaching responsibilities that trainee doctors should have at different stages of training and, as a consequence, the teaching skills that they need to learn.

Probity and health

Probity is a quality essential to good professional practice because patients depend upon the integrity of every doctor. Sickness hampers a doctor's ability to practise, both functionally and in terms of time lost. Whereas assessments of probity will be revealed in breaches rather than in observance, records of sick leave are the simplest way to demonstrate good health, although a failure to acknowledge mental ill-health can be a serious handicap.

Developing a content matrix

Principle 2, as defined by the PMETB, identifies the importance of a blueprint or test matrix, from which assessment should be drawn. This, it recommends, should be available to all stakeholders involved in the assessment system.

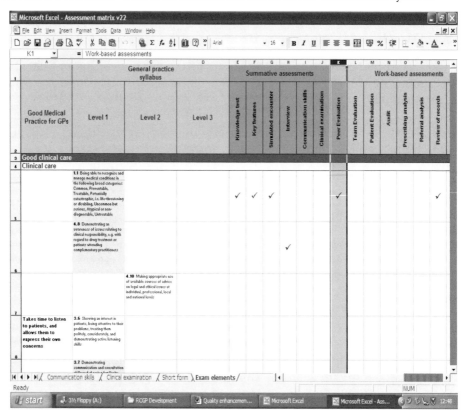

Figure 17.1 A section of the content matrix.

As an illustration of this, a small section of a content matrix developed by examiners for the MRCGP examination is shown in Figure 17.1. In this example, each element of the MRCGP examination syllabus is matched to *Good Medical Practice*.[9].

The content matrix enables individual elements of the MRCGP syllabus, which have a unique reference number, to be linked with an appropriate assessment. It also includes a third dimension: a timescale of when assessments could take place. The development of an assessment matrix therefore represents a critical step in the pathway to the selection of appropriate test methods.

Workplace assessment: tools, methods and sufficiency of evidence

What sort of evidence can we collect to chronicle the performance of a doctor within a workplace setting? Clinical outcomes might seem obvious criteria, and are used for some specific fields of practice, such as the performance of more experienced trainees at specialist registrar (SpR) grade in the craft specialities of medicine. The practice of medicine is largely a team activity and for the majority of doctors in training it can be difficult to relate a particular outcome to the performance of a specific trainee.

The hurdles that doctors in training must leap include the examinations set by the royal colleges (or other competent authorities in the case of general practice). Although these examinations will continue, their reliability and relevance to direct patient care has been challenged.[24,25,26] Work is being done to make these tests more pertinent to clinical practice and compatible with the run-through grade.

Although recording the numbers of cases or procedures undertaken does not describe the skill or accuracy with which work was done, it has been shown that the more tasks that are carried out satisfactorily, the greater the skill acquired and demonstrated by the performer. Practice makes perfect; it is both sensible and useful to keep records of the numbers of tasks performed and to employ them as part of the evidence that skill is advancing.

Experience of a variety of other methods of assessment has shown that there are three kinds of observations that seem to provide reliable, repeatable and consistent assessments of performance. These are the mini-clinical examination or mini-CEX; the structured case-based discussion; and the 360° appraisal based upon the criteria described in *Good Medical Practice*. These observations can be graded so that the progress of trainees and the development of improved skills can be charted. Furthermore, they are best performed in the workplace.

In primary care, general practitioners (GPs) have developed the use of video recordings of consultations as a tool for improving clinical practice.[27] In surgery, the design of effective task-based objective structured clinical examinations (OSCEs) is supporting the assessment of surgical skills.[28]

Mini-CEX

It has been traditional for clinical skills to be assessed by either the long case presentation or the short case examination. Recently, in a bid to marry reliability with economy of time, a version of the short case examination, popularly known as the 'mini-CEX', has become widely used in the USA. Each mini-CEX examines a specific clinical system or skill and the assessment is recorded in a standard format.

In order to enable the mini-CEX to be compatible with clinical practice, Norcini[17] evaluated reliability and reproducibility in the context of the number of mini-CEX observations made in a clinical placement. Each mini-CEX takes 15–20 minutes to complete and they can be performed in either an inpatient or outpatient setting. Between four and 12 mini-CEX evaluations are needed to demonstrate consistent results. Suitable times when a mini-CEX could be introduced for trainee assessment would be during the post-take ward round or as a planned exercise during a scheduled outpatient clinic.

Structured case-based discussion

When doctors are referred to the GMC because their practice is thought to be below an acceptable standard, one way in which their practice is evaluated under GMC performance procedures is through the use of the structured case-based discussion.[29] A case is chosen that is within the range of practice of the doctor whose performance is being evaluated, ideally one on which they have worked and the examiner prepares a set of reasonable questions covering the skills under test. A formal planning sheet is drawn up to include the questions and to allow the answers to be graded according to responses which were considered appropriate beforehand. The discussion takes place over a booked afternoon, when about 12 prepared cases are covered.

This format does not lend itself easily to the assessment of doctors in training. For most training posts, the cases that would be suitable for the assessment of a trainee in that post are predictable. With suitable preparation, it would be possible to cover a dozen appropriate cases in the three-month period and to do this as a coda to the post-take ward round.

360° appraisal (multi-source feedback)

Davies and colleagues[20] developed a workplace 360° assessment of performance which employs between 20 and 25 standards constructed to evaluate the performance of a doctor in training against the criteria described in *Good Medical Practice*. Typical criteria include 'Ability to diagnose patient problems', 'Appropriate utilisation of resources' and 'Verbal communication with colleagues'. Observers are allowed to leave out some questions if they feel that they are unable to rate a particular skill or attribute. Davies evaluated the reliability of these assessments with respect to numbers of observers and their areas of expertise, and found that seven observers give a reproducibility of less than one point on a seven-point rating scale. Analysis of the responses showed that while consultants were best able to rate clinical and diagnostic skills, nursing staff were the most able to assess technical ability.

Video recording

Visual records of consultation practice have proved useful in demonstrating to trainees the quality of their skills and in aiding improvement. The Royal College of General Practitioners (RCGP) has led the way in developing this tool, which is now an integral part of the learning experience of vocational trainees.

The video module of the current MRCGP examination is criterion-referenced and has proved to be an educational driver, in particular in enhancing patient-centred consulting skills.[27] It tests integrative skills, but, in common with other performance assessment methods, case-specificity is a problem and affects reliability. It could become a valuable part of formative assessment as a work-based method. Many have urged that video recordings be employed in the same way to support learning in outpatient settings in hospital, but progress has been slow, because of lack of funds and pressure of clinical work. It is hoped that this method will become a regular learning tool in secondary and tertiary practice, with the provision of more resources for teaching.

Task-based OSCE

Considerable strides have been made in developing model surgical scenarios in which the performance of trainee surgeons can be reliably measured against that of the expert surgeon. Professor Ara Darzi has pioneered this work in the UK and his general surgical OSCE can distinguish the new surgical senior house officer (SHO) from the average SpR and the consultant surgeon in terms of their relative skill.[28] Other models are in development, for example in surgery, and these have the potential to support the evaluation of surgical performance in theatre with reproducible and consistent data. Within general practice the rationale for the simulated patient encounter is derived from studies of the OSCE, which has been used as a method of allowing performance to be sampled across a range of patient problems. The method has been criticised for being reductionist and relying on binary judgements using a checklist approach that rewards proficiency rather than expertise. Although this aids reliability, the atomisation that occurs in the OSCE overlooks the integrative skills that doctors require. Efforts to overcome this have been made with modified OSCE examinations in which extra time is allowed for more complex aspects of patient problems to be assessed and for a structured oral examination.

An alternative approach is to use standardised patients rather than real patients, which provides consistency of presentation and the ability to control the choice of problems. This could enable assessment to be linked directly to learning objectives in a realistic clinical setting.[30] The advantage of this approach relates to greater reliability when compared with the variation of case specificity of workplace assessments such as the mini-CEX.

The current simulated surgery component of the MRCGP has shown acceptable and consistent reliability.[31]

Training in learning and assessing

Society needs to be confident that doctors are trained to an acceptable level of competence, and that they maintain their skills throughout their professional life, but the better education, training and validated assessment of doctors will cost time and money. Although the educational opportunities that are an integral part of service work must be seized, trainees will continue to need time set aside for learning in more formal environments. In the future, a greater proportion of the consultant contractual commitment must be allocated to teaching time if the aspirations of 'Modernising Medical Careers' (MMC) are to be delivered.[32] More money will be needed to pay for professional administrative and teaching staff to underpin the explicit requirements of the curriculum.

All trainees should complete the managing life course, or similar, before the award of the CCT. In the London Deanery it is planned to weave the components of managing life into the fabric of the foundation course, basic specialist training (BST) and higher specialist training (HST), so as to develop these important abilities while allowing the doctor in training increased responsibility in these areas.

Consultants will have to continue to shoulder increased responsibility for training their successors. However, few of them have been trained to teach, appraise and assess, although some do this very well while others are less effective. A significant investment must be made in courses to 'train the trainers' in order to improve the quality of clinical education. It may be that a few consultants will prove unable to teach effectively, but the assistance of the majority of all consultants will be needed if postgraduate medical education is to be modernised.

All prospective GP trainers within the London Deanery are already required to complete a 'teach the teachers' course satisfactorily; this is educationally accredited and leads to a postgraduate certificate in education.

Records

A key element of modern training and assessment is the requirement for accountability. Those reviewing the performance of a doctor who was assessed as competent, but who is later found to be incompetent, will need to know the grounds on which the original assessment was made. Consequently, it is vital that accurate records of the performance of all trainees are made and retained. These records may be paper, electronic or video recordings. Copies of the records should remain in the possession of trainers, while trainees keep the originals. A case can be made for additional copies to be held by the trust or the deanery, and some colleges already request copies of some assessments.

Every doctor in training will have a folder or portfolio containing the records of his or her achievements in training from medical school onwards. The folder will hold all relevant logbooks, appraisals and assessments, certificates of attendance at meetings and the information required for validation and revalidation by the GMC. It will hold 360° appraisal summaries, mini-CEX records and the reports of structured case-based discussions. Where video recordings of performances have been made, they should be included, together with the appraisals that followed them. The opportunistic way in which mini-CEX and structured case-based discussions may take place will require the development of standard recording sheets, so that assessments will be consistent from session to session as well as between trainees and across trust and deanery boundaries. Ultimately, appropriate information technology tools, possibly adapted for use in hand-held computers, will simplify and standardise this approach.

With respect to the development of workplace assessment in general practice, it is anticipated that the specific competencies that will need to be demonstrated, together with guidance relating to the assessment tools and the sufficiency of evidence required will be agreed nationally. This information will be made available to learners, teachers and assessors throughout the educational network.

Application to 'Modernising Medical Careers'

How should assessment be carried out in the new training pathways described in MMC?

Foundation course

The MMC policy requires that doctors completing the foundation course demonstrate appropriate competencies to enter BST. A combination of the mini-CEX, structured case-based discussions and 360° appraisal are suitable assessments. Certain specialities are keen that, where possible, experience gained during the foundation course should be included in accreditation. For example, the three-month initial anaesthetic training could be a part of a foundation course for trainees aiming at that discipline. Surgical experience could be assessed by a general surgical OSCE, because an objective assessment of surgical aptitude is a valuable observation.

All doctors in their second foundation year should have 'meaningful' experience in primary care. This is an ideal environment in which to learn core generalist skills, such as consultation skills, and could be assessed using the tools of observation, video recording and feedback, in which GPs are very experienced.

Basic specialist training and higher specialist training programmes

Experience in BST differs from foundation experience in two principal ways: clinical work being limited to a speciality, and undertaking more responsibility for outpatients. A structured approach to learning, more in line with the curriculum for HST, will be introduced by the colleges and appropriate modifications of the mini-CEX, structured case-based discussions and 360° appraisal will be employed.

Eight years of experience of SpR training in HST has taught a great deal about appraisal and assessment. Emphasis is on workplace assessment, not as a part of the RITA process, and this imperative will remain an integral part of the future management of postgraduate education.

Ultimately, the introduction of the run-through grade for a majority of specialities will mean that both teaching and training methods, and systems of assessment will be homologous for BST and HST.

Primary care training

It is anticipated that a period of three years' post-foundation training will be available, and teaching and learning will be directed towards a nationally agreed curriculum for general practice. The training programme will be competency-based and the competencies may be demonstrated 'when ready' by a combination of assessment methods likely to consist of workplace assessments, simulated clinical encounter testing (based on an OSCE format) and applied knowledge testing (machine-marked). Higher professional education (HPE) may be available for a further period of two years, followed by an optional period of additional training for those contemplating becoming general practitioners with special interests (GPSIs).

Ten key points

- Standard assessments of doctors in training will be introduced for all grades
- Assessments will conform to the principles described by the PMETB
- Assessments will be referenced to a curriculum derived from *Good Medical Practice*
- Assessments must be valid, reliable, evidence-based and cost-effective
- Assessments of relevant skills and competencies must match progress

- Systematic observation of clinical practice will be a core assessment
- A variety of records of performance will be made by multiple observers
- Standardised national methods of recording assessments will be used
- Trainers and trainees will be trained in assessing and being assessed
- Resources must be made available to permit these improvements.

References

1   Bolsin SN (1998) Professional misconduct in the Bristol case. *Med J Aus.* **169**: 369–72.

2   Horton R (2001) The real lesson from Harold Shipman. *Lancet.* **357**: 82–3.

3   Hunter M (2001) Alder Hey report condemns doctors, management and coroner. *BMJ.* **322**: 255.

4   Hart E and Hazelgrove J (2001) Understanding the organisational context for adverse events in the health services: the role of cultural censorship. *Quality in Health Care.* **10**: 257–62.

5   Dowling SM (2003) The metric of medical education validity: on the meaningful interpretation of assessment data. *Journal of Medical Education.* **37**: 830–7.

6   Jolly B and Grant J (1997) *The Good Assessment Guide.* London Joint Centre for Education in Medicine, Milton Keynes.

7   London Deanery *London Deanery Business Plan 2003/4.* London Deanery, London.

8   Southgate L and Grant J (2003). Principles and Standards for an Assessment System for Postgraduate Medical Training: Paper for the PMETB subgroup on assessment.

9   General Medical Council (2001) *Good Medical Practice.* GMC, London.

10 Gorter S, Rethans JJ, van der Heijde D *et al.* (2002) Reproducibility of clinical performance assessment in practice using incognito standardized patients. *Medical Education.* **36**: 827–32.

11 Prideaux D (2003) Curriculum design. *BMJ.* **326**: 268–70.

12 Harden R, Crosby J and Davis M (1991) Outcomes based education: Part 1 an introduction to outcomes-based education. *Medical Teacher.* **21**: 7–14.

13 Department of Health (2002) *Unfinished Business. Proposals for Reform of the Senior House Officer Grade.* DOH, London.

14 Miller G (1990) The assessment of clinical skills/competence/performance. *Academic Medicine.* **65**(suppl 40): S63–7.

15 Wilkinson J, Benjamin A and Wade W (2003) Assessing the performance of doctors in training. *BMJ.* **327**: s91–2.

16 Southgate L, Hays RB, Norcini J *et al.* (2001) Setting performance standards for medical practice: a theoretical framework. *Medical Education.* **35**: 474–81.

17 Norcini J (2003) ABC of learning and teaching in medicine. Work based assessment. *BMJ.* **326**: 753–5.

18 Swanson D, Clauser B and Case S (1999) Clinical skills assessment with standardized patients in high-stakes tests: A framework for thinking about score precision, equating, and security. *Adv Health Sci Educ Theory Pract.* **4**: 67–106.

19 Rethans J, Sturmans F, Drop M *et al.* (1991) Assessment of performance in actual practice of general practitioners by use of standardised patients. *Br J Gen Pract.* **41**: 97–9.

20 Archer J and Davies H (2004) Sheffield Peer Review Assessment Tool (SPRAT) for consultants: screening for poorly performing doctors. *Health Services Journal. in press.*

21 Kacperek L (1997) Non-verbal communication: the importance of listening. *British Journal of Nursing.* **6**, 275–9.

22 Hollander H and Loeser H (2002) Anticipatory quality improvement process for curricular reform. *Academic Medicine.* **77**: 930–5.

23 Heard S and Paice E (2002) Unfinished business – an opportunity for change. *Hospital Medicine.* **63**: 644–55.

24 Tamblyn R, Abrahamowicz M, Dauphinee WD *et al.* (2002) Association between licensure examination scores and practise in primary care. *JAMA.* **288**: 3019–26.

25 McManus IC, Moorey-Suner J, Dave JE *et al.* on behalf of the MRCP (UK) Part I Examination Board and the Federation of Royal Colleges of Physicians MRCP (UK) Central Office (2003) Junior doctors. Reliability of the Part I MRCP (UK) Examination, 1984–2001. *Journal of Medical Education.* **37**: 609–11.

26 Wass V, Wakeford R, Neighbour R *et al.* (2003) Achieving acceptable reliability in oral examinations: an analysis of the Royal College of General Practitioners membership examination's oral component. *Medical Education.* **37**:126–31.

27 Tate P, Foulkes J, Neighbour R *et al.* (1999) Assessing physicians' interpersonal skills via videotaped encounters: a new approach for the MRCGP. *Journal of Health Communication.* **4**: 143–52.

28 Moorthy K, Munoz, Y, Sarkar SK *et al.* (2003) Objective assessment of technical skills in surgery. *BMJ.* **327**: 1032–7.

29 Southgate L, Campbell M, Cox J *et al.* (2001) The General Medical Council's performance procedures: the development and implementation of tests of competence with examples from general practice. *Medical Education.* **35**: 20–8.

30 Polioli L (1995) Standardised patients: as we evaluate so shall we reap. *Lancet.* **345**: 966–8.

31 Burrows P and Bingham L (1999) The simulated surgery – an alternative to videotape submission for the consulting skills component of the MRCGP examination: the first year's experience. *Br J Gen Pract.* **49**: 269–72.

32 Department of Health (2003) *Modernising Medical Careers. The Response of the Four UK Health Ministers to the Consultation on Unfinished Business: Proposals for the Reform of the Senior House Officer Grade.* Department of Health, London. (www.mmc.nhs.uk/keyarticles/FINAL_VERSION_UK_POLICY_STA.PDF)

CHAPTER 18

Mentoring for doctors in primary and secondary care

Caroline Doherty and Owen Hanmer

Introduction

This chapter reflects on why mentoring is particularly important for doctors, explains the authors' approach to mentoring and describes the development of two major London Deanery-funded mentoring programmes: one for general practitioner (GP) non-principals in north-west London primary care, and the other for new consultants across five acute sector trusts in London. The chapter also identifies what makes an effective programme and offers the reader some of the outcomes of these mentoring programmes.

Why the London Deanery has been interested in developing mentoring programmes for doctors

Doctors often have great difficulty in seeing themselves as people in need. Their traditional culture has been one of self-reliance, clinical independence, and a resistance to personal management and close forms of supervision. However, like their colleagues in other disciplines, doctors need to make personal decisions about their lives and careers, often in the context of their work, and this may be difficult to do against a background of change and uncertainty beyond their control. Sources of informal support from colleagues within hospitals are disappearing and, increasingly, doctors are turning to mentors to help them reflect about personal issues, facilitate their decision-making and benefit from a supportive, reflective space.

Uncertainty arises from changes in training and working, and from the political, social and professional drivers for change. Newly qualified doctors now need to make an early decision about their future training and careers. Training programmes are being shortened, the nature of work as a trained specialist is changing and more doctors are seeking to train and work flexibly. The National Health Service (NHS) is undergoing change which is driven politically and by the changing expectations of patients and services. The workforce is becoming more diverse and concerned with the work–life balance and the changing roles and expectations of parents and carers. Continuing professional development (CPD) and clinical practice now require active lifelong learning, annual appraisal and revalidation.

In 1998 the Standing Committee on Postgraduate Medical and Dental Education (SCOPME) published a report, *Supporting Doctors and Dentists at Work: an inquiry into mentoring.*[1] This report recognised that mentoring could form a valuable part of a framework of support for doctors; that it should be entirely voluntary and confidential; and that support needs were likely to change at different stages of a medical career. It found that there was much to be gained from informal support from peers and other health professionals, but acknowledged the complementary role of formal systems and the importance of local ownership and development, of time away from the workplace, and the importance of training and support for mentors. It emphasised the positive, facilitative and developmental nature of mentoring and the separation from assessment or monitoring of performance. The report recommended that awareness of mentoring should be increased and opportunities be made widely available but not imposed.

It is important that support through mentoring is not confused with educational supervision and training, clinical supervision or clinical management. Mentoring does not seek to develop competences. It should take place outside work relationships and the workplace. It is not remedial and should not be used to address issues of performance. It should be seen as a separate but complementary process.

The important role of mentoring has been endorsed by the Department of Health, the medical royal colleges and faculties, and other professional bodies.[2,3,4,5]

Who benefits from mentoring?

Support for all doctors through mentoring is likely to be helpful at key times of career development and transition, for example when doctors make training and career decisions, take on new roles and responsibilities, return to work after career breaks or approach retirement.

There are also likely to be key groups of doctors who would benefit from this form of support. The London Deanery has already focused on developing programmes for specific groups such as GP non-principals or independent doctors and new consultants, and the very different needs and responses of these doctors are described below. There is also likely to be a role for mentoring in the support of women and doctors from ethnic minority communities working in specialities where they have been traditionally under-represented. The London Deanery is also actively exploring how mentoring can be made more widely available to trainees in the foundation programme and in specialist training programmes, as these are important times of transition when difficult career and life–work choices are made.

The London Deanery approach to mentoring

So what is this about?

The term 'mentoring' can be confusing and imprecise. Definitions vary according to organisational and professional context, and also to the intended outcomes or purpose of the mentoring. Even within medical settings mentoring can be defined very differently, as has been highlighted by the recent report, *Mentoring for Doctors: Enhancing the Benefit.*[5]

This confusion about what mentoring is can be further compounded by some similar confusion around other one-to-one development processes, such as appraisal, clinical supervision, coaching and counselling. These terms are often used interchangeably for any supportive one-to-one developmental work. So, in all this potential confusion it has been particularly important to describe how mentoring is defined in deanery-led programmes – starting with what mentoring is *not*.

As most people know, the traditional view of mentoring developed in Western culture from the ancient Greek story of how Odysseus left his son in the care of an older wise man, Mentor, as he set out on his legendary journey. The term 'mentor' then became associated with someone who was seen as 'a wise and trusted adviser'. Traditionally, in organisations and the professions, a mentor was an older or more senior colleague (usually a man) who would take a more junior colleague (also usually a man) under his wing and advise and support him as his career developed. This was often a relationship based on patronage – wherin a mentee or protégé could expect his mentor, because of his position in the company or profession, to 'open doors' for him.

However, in recent years, the concept of patronage, which lies at the heart of this traditional approach, has become much less valued and acceptable within the public sector because of its capacity to exclude sections of the community and workforce. In particular, in medicine, women and people from minority ethnic communities have had less access to powerful patrons who could support their career development

Consequently, over the past decade there has been a move towards making mentoring within medicine a more open and accessible process. The model itself has evolved. The London Deanery mentoring programmes in both primary and secondary care now promote a 'developmental mentoring' model, which has some significant differences from the traditional model rooted in Greek mythology.

The key ingredients of the developmental mentoring approach include:

- a finite relationship: the deanery programmes have offered mentees between four and six mentoring sessions over a period of 12–18 months
- personal support: where the mentor offers a supportive one-to-one relationship; this, of course, is the heart of mentoring
- a focus on professional and career development at a point of change or transition – where the mentee looks towards planning for the future or making sense of a new situation
- a reflective space: time to think, develop insights and learn from experience
- a mentee-centred approach – in which the mentee sets the agenda and the mentor agrees to support and empower.

For mentees, working well with a mentor within the developmental mentoring model involves taking responsibility for one's own development. It may also mean 'owning up' to vulnerabilities, acknowledging and sharing problems, ambitions and fears. It can be a challenging process and to be successful there needs to be a confidential and trusting relationship.

The task for the mentor within the developmental mentoring approach is, therefore, to:

- facilitate reflection, learning and development, rather than acting as an expert or teacher
- support self-directed learning – encouraging mentees to be responsible for identifying their own development needs and finding ways to address them
- stay mentee-centred in approach – focusing on the mentee and what he or she needs from a session and the relationship
- act as a signpost – offering information when it is appropriate, as opposed to giving advice or telling mentees what to do.

For both mentors and mentees, working within this developmental mentoring model often has meant learning to work in a different paradigm from the traditional medical model (Table 18.1).

This approach to mentoring involves mentors stepping outside the role of the 'experienced expert' – the knowledgeable and respected GP or consultant – and stepping back into a more supportive role and encouraging mentees to find their own expert and expertise. Developmental mentoring therefore represents a significant challenge to many of the norms of medical culture: it may not be for everyone, so who becomes involved and why?

Table 18.1: Mentoring – a paradigm shift for doctors?

The medical approach	The mentoring approach
The context: • 10 minute consultations The skills and approach: • Listening and asking questions to diagnose and problem-solve Underpinning beliefs: • Doctor as expert • Patients need curing and fixing	The context: • 90-minute mentoring sessions The skills and approach: • Listening and asking questions to understand, enable and facilitate insight Underpinning beliefs: • Mentee as own expert • Mentees can find own solutions and ways forward given a supportive framework
Values: • Formal education, training and success in exams • Competitive culture – not sharing your feelings • Programmed knowledge and single-loop learning • Learning from experts – being right and having answers • Intellectual intelligence • Traditionally masculine	Values: • Learning to learn, learning about yourself, taking risks, experimenting • Collaborative and supportive culture – where feelings are acceptable • Finding your own solutions, double- and triple-loop learning • Learning from experience • Emotional intelligence • Traditionally feminine

The mentors

Deanery programmes have recruited experienced GPs and consultants to act as mentors for their peers. When defining how much experience is relevant, the London Deanery has taken a pragmatic view that mentors need enough experience to be credible to colleagues, but it recognises that in some situations too wide a seniority gap may (but not always) be a hindrance. In practice, the majority of those who have come forward to become mentors have been GPs or consultants, mostly in their mid-career. They tend to have a minimum of five years' experience at a senior level. The motivation to become a mentor varies: some are keen to develop another dimension of their career; many have been active in training and education and have an active interest in supporting colleagues; some felt very unsupported as juniors and wish to change that situation for future generations.

All mentors on the London Deanery mentoring programmes prepare for the role by participating in a two-day workshop and they are supported once they start mentoring, via quarterly learning set meetings. The mentor preparation workshops focus on developing understanding of the role and the mentoring approach and on refining intervention styles. For most doctors, the most challenging part of learning to become an effective mentor lies in learning to listen and ask questions in order to facilitate reflection ('active listening') rather than listening and asking questions in order to diagnose and problem-solve – it can be hard to switch off the medical model!

Becoming a mentor has provided significant career enrichment opportunities for many mentors. It has been the catalyst for moving into other education or training roles, and many GP mentors have become GP appraisers.

The mentees

The Deanery programmes targeted GP non-principals or independent GPs in primary care and new consultants in the secondary sector. In primary care the mentees, in dialogue with the deanery, identified themselves as being isolated and unsupported at a period of significant service and professional change. Many were at a point of career uncertainty and potential change: deciding to become a GP principal, returning to work, balancing work and carer responsibilities or heading towards retirement. For example, they said they wanted to have a mentor to look at areas such as:

'Learning more about becoming a partner'
'Personal development'
'Juggling/prioritising work with a young family and a medical husband'
'Developing PDPs'
'Consolidating training into real life and part-time general practice whilst building confidence and self esteem'
'Getting things "in order" for applying for a part-time principal post'
'Lost confidence having limited time for career – due to family commitments'

Those who participated were actively seeking support. The programme developed a respected profile so the uptake was relatively high. Over three years the mentoring programme supported nearly 100 GPs.

It was different, however, in the secondary sector. The programmes in hospital trusts were designed to provide a level of 'preventive' support to new consultants as they made the transition into a first consultant post. They were established as a result of recognising that many new consultants were finding this transition particularly stressful, and some in particular were feeling unprepared for the leadership and management side of their new role.

Those who applied for a mentor through the programme identified a range of needs, such as:

'Advice and guidance through transition from trainee to consultant'
'People management'
'Relationships with colleagues (many of whom have been their seniors)'
'Achieving change at work'

'Balancing work commitments with home life'

'Career development'

'Am early in my career and would value the input/support of a mentor in shaping my career and dealing with unfamiliar roles'

'To become more confident and effective in my role – reduction on stress and uncertainty'

'Management of the team and juniors'

'Stress management'

At the time of writing these programmes are all still in their relatively early stages but the indication is that the uptake of mentee places is slow. It seems that many new consultants may not yet recognise the value and potential of developmental mentoring support in the same way that GPs have done.

Why this might be so raises a number of questions and speculations. Do new consultants understand what developmental mentoring is and how it may be helpful to them? Is asking for any sort of support culturally still taboo for consultants? Is there still a fear that it will (or may be) seen as a sign of weakness and potential failure? Are the levels of trust needed to sustain a mentoring programme within hospital trusts sufficiently robust to allow new consultants to feel confident about confidentiality? Have the mentoring programmes recruited consultant mentors who are credible to the potential mentees? Is mentoring the most appropriate model to address the needs of new consultants at this early career stage – or might they need more formal education or training programmes on the development of leadership and professionalism? All these questions will need to be addressed in the review and evaluation of the programmes.

Developing effective mentoring programmes

What has been learnt?

Developing these programmes over the past four years, a range of factors that can help or hinder a successful programme has been identified. Some of these are universal to all mentoring programmes, but some are more pertinent in either a primary or secondary care setting.

Key factors in building successful mentoring programmes

Stakeholder involvement in planning

At its most simple level, all those who are essential to the success of the programme need to have an input into the planning. For example, in the secondary care sector, programmes are most likely to be effective when the senior management and senior doctors give a programme high-profile support by promoting its value and providing resources, when experienced and credible colleagues participate as mentors and most importantly when potential mentees recognise their development needs and actively look for support. This takes time and can feel frustrating, but without good foundations the effect of the programme will be limited.

Programmes need a clear overall framework

Mentors and mentees need to be clear about the expectations and nature of the relationship from the start. Both primary and secondary care programmes promote mentoring as a 'formal and finite relationship'. 'Formal' means it has an agreed purpose and is part of a managed process. It is not a friendship (but it will be friendly and supportive as well as challenging). The 'finite' nature helps to focus mentees' development, and in not creating dependency.

Assured confidentiality

Confidentiality is essential for all the obvious reasons of trust and credibility. Limitations to confidentiality, such as concerns in maintaining responsibilities under the General Medical Council (GMC) duties of a doctor and any trust policies, need to be clearly explained at the outset of the relationship and systems for dealing with concerns need to be in place.

Choice in matching

Developing a constructive and supportive relationship is a very personal thing. It is often hard to predict how people will get on so offering a choice of mentors, with an option to change if the initial choice proves not to be suitable is essential. This can be difficult to manage where there is a small pool of mentors. The London Deanery programmes have operated a 'guided choice' system, whereby two or three possible mentors are identified and mentees choose from these.

In making matches in secondary care the London Deanery has sought to match away from speciality and to offer a mentor who has no investment in the mentees' day-to-day work. In primary care the same principles have held but matching concerns have often centred on geography – trying to strike a balance between someone not in the same area and not having to travel too far to meet.

Active administration

This may seem minor but programmes do need to have someone who maintains an overview, keeps in touch with matched pairs and, where necessary, will 'chase' and remind mentees and mentors about their commitment to meet, etc. In 2002, Klaseen and Clutterbuck[6] identified this as a key and often overlooked role, without which programmes tend to fade after the initial enthusiasm of the first year.

Role preparation

Mentors and mentees both benefit from being prepared for their roles. The London Deanery programmes have run very successful two-day mentor preparation workshops for mentors, but have been less systematic about preparing mentees to understand the mentoring process and how to get the most from it. This is an area for development – feedback from both mentors and mentees indicates that many start the process unclear about how to use it. Many potential mentees may not start the process at all because they do not understand it!

Systems for support and problem-solving

Mentors value access to ongoing support. Programmes have quarterly learning set meetings, usually a lunchtime meeting, at which mentors can reflect on issues arising from sessions. In addition, it is important to have access to more immediate back-up should problems arise. It is also helpful for mentors to have e-group contact to share information about resources, etc., which may be useful for their mentees.

Sufficient resources

As ever, the appropriate resources are often critical to the success of mentoring programmes. This problem has been addressed differently across the sectors. In primary care the programme has paid mentors a small fee for each mentoring session, as well as paying the locum costs for the training and learning sets. Mentees are not paid. In the secondary sector consultant mentoring has been built into job plans and has been seen as a legitimate use of flexible sessions, but time as always is an issue.

Realistic timescales

It takes longer to establish a programme than you may think. Programmes need a minimum of two years to become established and provide mentoring to a cohort of mentees.

Outcomes – what do doctors gain from mentoring?

There is a small but growing evidence base that mentoring provides doctors with a range of valued outcomes.[5] Feedback from the London Deanery mentoring programmes supports this and shows gains for both mentors and mentees at a number of levels. As with many other learning and development activities, it is often difficult to make a direct cause and effect connection between mentoring and changed behaviour. However, it is clear that for most mentees and many mentors their involvement in mentoring is often a catalyst for some change and professional development.

Outcomes for mentees

In the feedback from a number of mentoring programmes, mentees consistently report what they get from the mentoring process in terms of support and self esteem:

'Confidence in my own ability and integrity'
'Self-confidence and an idea of self-worth'
'Regained self-esteem and self-confidence in my value system, which had been questioned and criticised'

In terms of career decisions:

'Decided to start training as a breast clinician'
'Have started as GP retainer'

In terms of insights and increased self-awareness:

'I talk too much'
'I am driven to get things right and to be liked'
'Need to improve communication'
'Greater insight into what I do and how I do it'

and, finally, in terms of impact on practice
'Improved my listening skills'
'Improved my consultation skills'
'Changed my consultation times'
'Able to be more assertive'.

Outcomes for mentors

Klasen and Clutterbuck[6] describe mentoring as a 'developmental conversation' that has the potential to create opportunities for learning and development for both mentors and mentees. This has been supported by the experiences of mentors on all London Deanery mentoring programmes. Overall, they found the experience both rewarding and motivating.

Mentors identified outcomes for themselves in terms of: increased self-awareness:

'That I tend to be too supportive and not challenging enough'
'I learnt about my own strengths and weaknesses and insight to myself as a person'

'I need to improve my communication'
'Perhaps I too have needs to be fulfilled in a professional relationship'
'Mentoring made me feel more positive about myself'.

Career development/career enrichment:

'I am now going to become an appraiser'
'Has given me status in my practice – now becoming a trainer'
'It feels good to be able to support a colleague'.

Insight into the organisation and service beyond their own direct experience:

'Better understanding of problems at the beginning of my career, which I learnt the hard way – wish mentoring was available when I joined general practice'
'Greater insight into what I do and why I do it'
'I am more aware of colleagues and their professional development'.

Outcomes for the organisation and service

It is hard to be confident in making claims about the impact of mentoring beyond individuals' experiences of personal and professional changes. There is some anecdotal evidence that indicates that access to mentoring support at critical career stages does help many doctors to stay engaged and to find their place in medicine. This can be particularly significant for parents and carers who may be struggling to maintain a work–home balance. So, it is not unreasonable to claim that mentoring can play an important role in the retention of some groups of doctors.

However, ensuring that doctors (and other healthcare professionals) have access to skilled mentoring support at times when they need it clearly plays an important part in creating a culture of support and lifelong learning. It helps to demonstrate the importance of caring for the professional carers in the NHS in order to provide a high-quality service to patients.

Ways forward

Awareness and interest in mentoring are increasing, and the available evidence base is currently being reviewed and published by the Improving Working Lives Doctors' Forum. However, six years have passed since SCOPME published its recommendations[1] and there is still much to do if support through mentoring is to be available and accessible to doctors in training and those taking on new responsibilities and roles. There are some clear steps that need to be taken that may help achieve this, as follows.

- Stakeholders need to do more to increase awareness and understanding, and to assess the potential need for mentoring.
- Stakeholders need to develop a strategy and framework for implementation that is clear, flexible, achievable and shared by them all.
- NHS trusts need to explore how mentors can be recruited and trained locally, recognise opportunities for joint training in generic skills and competences, and the need for a small initial pool of mentors to act as the nucleus for a developing programme.
- Deaneries, medical royal colleges and faculties need to explore how they can provide mentoring to key groups of doctors who would benefit from this form of support.
- Trainees and other potential mentees need to become involved in the development and evaluation of mentoring processes, and to develop a sense of shared ownership.
- Evidence of good practice and effectiveness needs to be reviewed, widely disseminated and appreciated, and implemented.

Conclusion

That mentoring makes a positive difference to the professional development and well-being of doctors is obvious from experience of the London Deanery programmes to date. However, mentoring programmes take time and resources to develop and without some dedicated support or resource, in a culture where asking for support is still not common, they tend to become a low priority. These positive benefits need to be more widely communicated in order to ensure that mentoring is widely available to all those who might benefit from it.

References

1 Standing Committee on Postgraduate Medical and Dental Education (1998) *Supporting Doctors and Dentists at Work: an inquiry into mentoring.* SCOPME, London.

2 Department of Health (2000) *The NHS Plan – A Plan for Investment, A Plan for Reform.* Department of Health, London.

3 Department of Health (2000) *International Recruitment of Consultants and General Practitioners for the NHS in England.* Department of Health, London.

4 Department of Health (2002) *Improving Working Lives for Doctors.* Department of Health, London.

5 Improving Working Lives Doctors' Forum (2004) *Mentoring for Doctors: enhancing the benefit.* Department of Health, London.

6 Klaseen N and Clutterbuck D (2002) *Implementing Mentoring Schemes.* Butterworth–Heinemann, Oxford.

CHAPTER 19

Lifelong learning in the NHS

Rhamesh Bhatt, Anne Hastie and Neil Jackson

Introduction

Government Health Policy[1] has highlighted the entitlement of all patients in the National Health Service (NHS) to receive high-quality care. Within its 10-year modernisation programme the Government has also stated clearly the need to ensure fair access to high-quality care wherever a patient is treated in the NHS.

In order to ensure the delivery of national quality standards, the Government has cited three key principles that will underpin these standards. These are:

- within local practice by a system of clinical governance
- through extended lifelong learning to ensure that NHS staff are equipped to maintain and develop their skills and expertise
- through modernised professional self-regulation.

This chapter will focus on the principle of lifelong learning and continuing professional development (CPD) in the NHS and its contribution to the quality agenda.

Continuing professional development and lifelong learning

Much emphasis is placed on what a doctor needs to do to become a registered specialist or general practitioner (GP). Criteria are set for acceptance on training programmes: these programmes must meet curricula set by training authorities, and they should include a robust assessment process. But all this happens within the first 10 years of a doctor's career, with the 'apprentice' model at the centre of postgraduate training. However, doctors may then go on to practice for more than 30 years without any need for further formal assessment of their skills or knowledge required to practise up-to-date medicine. The General Medical Council (GMC) booklet, *Good Medical Practice*[2] sets out the basic principles of good practice and is the basis for many training and developmental activities. It includes three brief two-sentence paragraphs on 'Keeping Up to Date', but, as the introduction to the booklet states, 'It is guidance and is not a set of rules nor is it exhaustive'.

Until recently, there was no onus on doctors to demonstrate their retention of skills and knowledge, or their acquisition of relevant new knowledge or skills. But there has been a change. Periodic revalidation by the GMC for all UK doctors will shortly be implemented across the UK.[3] All doctors in primary and secondary care now have to demonstrate continuing professional development (CPD) activity within an appraisal process based on the main headings of *Good Medical Practice* (*see* www.gmc-uk.org/revalidation/index.html) in the countries of the UK. It is anticipated that satisfactory annual cycle of peer review of CPD via appraisals will lead to revalidation every five years.[4]

This change of approach in revalidation and being able to demonstrate retention of skills and knowledge[5] has been prompted in part by the inquiries into some of the very public failings of medical care; for example, the inquiry into the deaths of children at Bristol Royal Infirmary. But there are compelling reasons why it is reasonable in a field such as medical care to require that practitioners continue to learn and demonstrate retentions of relevant skills. In 1988 the American College of Physicians estimated that 85% of all prescriptions written by doctors who had graduated in 1960 'will be for a drug about which they will have received little formal education'.[6] Moreover, significant changes in the indication of use of drugs may evolve over time; for example, opinion on the appropriacy of hormone replacement therapy (HRT) has altered as information from long-term follow-up of women on HRT has become available. Of course innovation is not confined to drugs. Considerable changes in surgical and diagnostic techniques and technologies have altered the ways many conditions are detected, investigated and treated. The incidence of disease may change and occasionally a new condition emerges; for example, all doctors who finished their postgraduate training before 1988 have learnt about HIV or AIDS through the process of CPD. Demographic changes, leading to increased survival of an ageing population in a technologically competent world, has seen an increase in the prevalence of chronic diseases, and demands a radical rethink in models of chronic disease management – requiring not just shifting significant proportions of such structured delivery into primary care with ensuing remodelling of care provided by GPs.[7] This shift will have a significant effect on skill mixes and the acquisition of new skills for GPs (and for the GP with special interest, GPwSI) and how doctors work with other healthcare practitioners, such as nurses with special interests, healthcare assistants and primary care managers. It will require GPs to learn to work in teams and in a more structured environment, with greater accountability through the process of clinical governance and increasing emphasis on quality.[8]

As well as clinical knowledge and skills, doctors need to be aware of the changing ideas and values of an evolving society, and should be competent to manage changes in public and patient expectations. For example, the scandal of the retention of organs at the Alder Hey Children's Hospital demonstrates a practice once routine throughout the NHS, which is now considered unacceptable. Such events have resulted in a robust response by the UK Government via the Chief Medical Officer (CMO) for England,[9] which highlights the issue of poor performance and proposes a regular cycle of appraisals for doctors.

It is clear that, in order to continue to practise safely and appropriately, doctors in all branches of medicine must be committed to a programme of CPD and of lifelong learning. In this chapter we will briefly discuss some of the terminology, examine the effectiveness of different approaches to continuing development and describe how this is played out in practice.

Lifelong learning

With such a challenging and all-encompassing agenda, going as it does beyond the doctors' role as a problem solver who uses specialised scientific knowledge, how do doctors, the rational, technical professionals[10] keep abreast of specialised scientific knowledge, respond to the changing normal and values of the wider society that affect scientific practice, provide an ever-increasing range of healthcare and remain refreshed? As a myriad of demands bear down upon them, one certainty is that doctors will need to be lifelong learners: to understand that learning and development does not stop at graduation nor at becoming a GP or a consultant in a speciality. From here on in, the traditional 'chalk and talk' and the apprenticeship ends abruptly; the doctor becomes the autonomous practitioner, the self-directed, adult learner,[11] who takes charge of his or her own learning. The current narrative of lifelong learning exhorts the virtues of every aspect of professional practice as a learning opportunity. It challenges the traditional distinction between formal and informal learning, and institutional contexts.[12] Indeed, medical practice lends itself well to experiential learning, whether this occurs in the consulting room (listening to patients), from colleagues and peers, in the operating theatre, in the emergency room or in a debate on the ethics of *in vitro* fertilisation. This richness of learning opportunity in the workplace and elsewhere provides the very raw material of CPD:

> A process of lifelong learning for all individuals and teams which enables professionals to expand and fulfil potential and which also meets the needs of patients and delivers the health and healthcare priorities of the NHS.[13]

Learning is, therefore, a continuing process throughout the professional life of doctors. Professional and personal development occurs through this learning. Adult learners reflect on experience in the workplace as well as other healthcare imperatives to identify learning needs that drives their learning and development. A review by the Chief Medical Officer[13] highlighted the need for improvement in quality through CPD and accepted the fundamentals of CPD: knowledge, skills and 'best professional attitudes'. The purpose of CPD is seen as helping doctors to meet the challenges of changes in healthcare, to encourage more reflection on practice and learning needs, and to make the educational methods used in practice more effective. CPD is seen as a key to delivering lifelong learning and some of the difficulties of measurement of effectiveness of CPD programmes is acknowledged. The emphasis is on learning styles and activities that are based on assessed learning needs; on the learning process rather than learning methods. The review[12] reinforced the move away from the formal, institutional and didactic to the lifelong learning process. As has been said of CPD: '... we are all doing it. Much of CPD is the recognition of learning we already do. Few innovations in my practice have come from attendance at a lecture – the traditional form of CME.'[14]

Effectiveness of CPD

The ultimate test of effectiveness of interventions which are included in the descriptions of CPD or lifelong learning in medical care is their effect on healthcare outcomes. A review of 50 randomised controlled trials in 1992 concluded that 'Broadly defined CME interventions using practice-enabling or reinforcing strategies consistently improve physician performance and, in some instances, healthcare outcomes.'[15]

In general practice

In primary care, the annual appraisal of GPs began in April 2003. This appraisal 'is a positive and developmental process for individual clinicians ... to give GPs feedback on their past performance, to chart their continuing progress and to identify development needs'.[16] This process encourages the use of many tools of lifelong learning. For example, through the use of a personal development plan (PDP), the process requires doctors to identify education and training needs, and set objectives, describe how these will be addressed and encourages participation in and review of these objectives. It is based on the sound principles of the 'learning cycle' whereby the learner moves through four stages of a cycle:

- concrete experience: clinical practice
- reflecting on the experience
- conceptualisation of learning needs
- active experimentation.

This learning activity is undertaken to meet identified needs.[17] The appraisal process is professionally led and peer-reviewed: the peers or the appraisers have received formal training for conducting such reviews on a one-to-one basis. The outcome is an agreed personal development plan (PDP) based on doctors' individual learning and development needs, with clearly identified learning objectives and action that the appraisee agrees to undertake, usually within an annual timeframe. The appraisee is encouraged to reflect on clinical practice under the main headings of *Good Medical Practice*,[2] and on the needs of the organisation and healthcare priorities set out nationally, such as national service frameworks and the new general medical services contract for GPs.[18] In addition, appraisees are asked to consider educational activities that are appropriate to the learning objectives, and which suit the learning style of the learner, and to consider a selection of learning and teaching methods. The emphasis is on moving away from the didactic lecture setting to active learning. Appraisees will capture the learning outcome in an educational portfolio and by instruments such as a reflective diary.

April 2004 saw the passing of the Postgraduate Educational Allowance (PGEA)[18] and thus the demise of accrediting attendance at educational meetings for GPs. The new paradigm of lifelong learning will, from now on, be enshrined in the PDP based on assessed learning needs, constructed in a spirit of personal and professional development, helped by a trained peer, reviewed annually and supported by the deanery (GP) tutor. GPs will thus reflect on practice[19] and record their learning outcomes in a growing educational portfolio.[20,21] If managed with confidence and resourced adequately, this will be a new dawn for the lifelong learners in the new NHS.

Prolonged study leave for general practitioners

In recent years GPs have been experiencing high levels of stress and low morale[22,23] resulting in a trend towards early retirement and part-time working.[24] Increasing numbers of GPs are indicating their intention to abandon direct patient care, with low job satisfaction being identified as a major factor for this.[25] Prolonged study leave (PSL) gives GPs an opportunity for refreshment by spending some time away from their service commitments in order to undertake a period of educational activity.[26] GPs can broaden their experience by studying for a higher degree, enhancing their role through the development of specialist medical knowledge or academic research. PSL can be undertaken on a full- or part-time basis up to a maximum of 260 working days, with the individual doctor receiving locum and educational allowances, which provide a contribution towards their overall expenses.

The opportunity to undertake PSL on a part-time basis was introduced in the mid-1990s, and has become an increasingly popular choice, suggesting that it is a welcome improvement to the regulations.[27] However, the uptake of PSL remains low, with a national annual rate of 0.77%,[28] and this may reflect difficulty in finding locums or resistance from other partners in the practice. Kemple[29] recommends careful advanced planning within a partnership to avoid such obstacles. Applications for PSL are sent to the Director of Postgraduate General Practice Education (DPGPE) for educational approval and must have prior agreement from the practice partners and the primary care trust (PCT). Applicants need to demonstrate in a written report that their period of PSL will benefit themselves, their practice, the PCT and the NHS as a whole.

Changes in the funding stream for PSL were introduced by the Department of Health in April 2004, when funding for both personal medical services (PMS) and general medical services (GMS) GPs became the responsibility of PCTs. Individual PCTs must determine whether the payment of funds to a GP for PSL is affordable, with regard to the PCT's budgetary targets for the year. This may result in a GP in one PCT being granted PSL funding, whereas a GP in another PCT is refused even though their proposal may be equally excellent.

The majority of GPs who undertake PSL find it a positive experience and return to their work in general practice[27] suggesting PSL may have a positive effect on GP retention. In addition, many of these GPs take on new responsibilities in fields important to the development of primary care.[27] The cost to the NHS of one doctor taking one year of full-time PSL (260 days) in the financial year 2004/2005 was £54 522, so it is important that positive outcomes can be demonstrated.

References

1 Secretary of State for Health (1998) *A First Class Service – Quality in the New NHS*. HMSO, London.

2 General Medical Council (2001) *Good Medical Practice*. GMC, London.

3 General Medical Council (2000) *Revalidation for Doctors: ensuring standards, securing the future*. GMC, London. (www.revalidationuk.info)

4 General Medical Council (2003) *A Licence to Practise and Revalidation*. GMC, London.

5 General Medical Council (2001) *Maintaining Good Medical Practice*. GMC, London.

6 Health and Public Policy Committee, American College of Physicians (1988) Improving medical education in therapeutics. *Ann Int Med.* **108**: 145–7.

7 Department of Health (2002) *The New GMS Contract*. DoH, London.

8 Secretary of State for Health (1998) *A First Class Service*. DoH, London.

9 Chief Medical Officer (2001) *Supporting Doctors, Protecting Patients*. DoH, London.

10 Schon D (1983) *The Reflective Practitioner*. Basic Books, New York.

11 Knowles M (1990) *The Adult Learner, A Neglected Species*. Texas Gulf, Houston, TX.

12 Harrison R, Reeve F, Hanson A and Clarke J (eds) (2002) *Supporting Life Long Learning* (Vol. 1). Oxford University Press, Oxford.

13 Chief Medical Officer (1998) *A Review of CPD in General Practice.* DoH, London.

14 Pringle M (2000) Foreword. In: Rughani A *The GP's Guide to Professional Development Plans.* Radcliffe Medical Press, Oxford.

15 Davis DA, Thomson MA, Oxman AD *et al.* (1992) Evidence for the effectiveness of CMW. *JAMA.* **268**: 1111–17.

16 Chief Medical Officer (2001) *Appraisals for General Practitioners.* DoH, London.

17 Kolb D (1985) *Experiential Learning: experience as a source of learning and development.* Prentice Hall, New Jersey.

18 Department of Health (2002) *The New GMS Contract.* DoH, London.

19 Burton J and Jackson N (2003) *Work-based Learning in Primary Care.* Radcliffe Medical Press, Oxford.

20 Royal College of General Practitioners (1993) *Portfolio-based Learning in General Practice.* Occasional Paper No 63. RCGP, London.

21 Pietroni R (2001) *The Toolbox for Portfolio Development.* Radcliffe Medical Press, Oxford.

22 Chambers R and Maxwell R (1989) Helping sick doctors. *BMJ.* **312**: 722–3.

23 Firth-Cozens J (1997) Predicting stress in general practitioners: 10 year follow up of postal survey. *BMJ.* **315**: 34–5.

24 Taylor DH and Leese B (1997) Recruitment, retention and time commitment change of general practitioners in England and Wales 1990–94: a retrospective study. *BMJ.* **314**: 1806–10.

25 Sibbal S, Bojke C and Gravelle H (2003) National survey of job satisfaction and retirement intentions among general practitioners in England. *BMJ.* **326**: 22–4.

26 NHS (1990) *Statement of Fees and Allowances.* **50.1.18**: 145–7.

27 Hastie A and Clark R (2004) An assessment of prolonged study leave. *Education for Primary Care.* **15**: 378–82.

28 Evans A, Ford J and Bahrami J (2002) Prolonged study leave: who takes it, and what is it for? *Education for Primary Care.* **13**: 451–6.

29 Kemple T (1998) Taking a sabbatical in general practice. *BMJ.* **316**: 2–3.

CHAPTER 20

General practitioners with a special interest

Imtiaz Gulamali and Neil Jackson

Introduction

In the process of modernising the National Health Service (NHS) it remains crucial to develop its workforce. For general practitioners (GPs), nurses and allied health professionals working in primary care, developing their roles will enable more patients to be managed out of hospital and away from the secondary care sector. In addition, by facilitating the process of developing an integrated approach to services across specialities and the primary and secondary care interface, patients will experience improved access to specialist services in the community, where previously they would have been referred to secondary care.

Developing the roles of primary healthcare staff can also enhance the management of chronic disease in the primary care setting. One such role is that of the GP with a special interest (GPwSI), who is first and foremost a generalist, but who is capable of delivering a clinical service beyond the scope of conventional general practice and who can receive referrals from other GPs in the primary care setting.

This chapter explores the developing GPwSI role and its many ramifications, including the reconfiguration of service provision for patients in primary care.

What is a general practitioner?

Before attempting to understand what we mean by a GP with a special interest, we need to know what a GP actually is. The definition of a GP varies from time to time as their role changes and develops. However, the latest consensus statement from the World Organization of Family Doctors (WONCA) defines a GP as:

> General practitioners/family doctors are specialist physicians trained in the principles of the discipline. They are personal doctors, primarily responsible

for the provision of comprehensive and continuing care to every individual seeking medical care irrespective of age, sex, and illness. They care for individuals in the context of their family, their community, and their culture, always respecting the autonomy of their patients. They recognize they will also have a professional responsibility to their community. In negotiating management plans with their patients they integrate physical, psychological, social, cultural, and existential factors, utilizing the knowledge and trust engendered by repeated contacts. General practitioners exercise their professional role by promoting health, preventing disease, and providing cure, care, or palliation. This is done either directly or through the services of others according to their health needs and resources available within the community they serve, assisting patients where necessary in accessing these services. They must take responsibility for developing and maintaining their skills, personal balance and values as a basis for effective and safe patient care.[1]

General practice is an academic and scientific discipline with its own educational content, research, evidence base and clinical activity. It is a clinical speciality, oriented to primary care, and GPs are specialist physicians trained in the principles of this discipline. A definition of the discipline of general practice must lead directly to the core competencies of general practice. 'Core' means essential to the discipline, irrespective of the healthcare system in which they are applied.

The central characteristics that define the discipline relate to abilities that every GP should master. They can be clustered into six core competencies:

- primary care management
- person-centred care
- specific problem-solving skills
- comprehensive approach
- community orientation
- holistic modelling.

To practise the speciality, the competent practitioner implements these competencies in three areas:

- clinical tasks
- communication with patients
- management of the practice.

As a person-centred scientific discipline, three background features should be considered as fundamental:

- Contextual: usually the context of the person, the family, the community and their culture

- Attitudinal: based upon on the doctor's professional capabilities, values and ethics
- Scientific: adopting a critical and research-based approach to practice and maintaining this through continuing learning and quality improvement.

The interrelation of core competencies, implementation areas and fundamental features characterise the discipline and underline the complexity of the speciality. Reform of national health systems is a common feature in the UK, as elsewhere in the world. Given changes in demography, medical advances, health economics and patients' needs and expectations, new ways of providing and delivering healthcare are being sought. It is perceived by policymakers that the traditional models of primary and secondary care are failing to meet the needs of the patients as well as the profession. Hence the development of the intermediate-level specialist (the GPwSI) to increase access at allocation close to the patient while giving support to the wider primary health community.[2]

Historical background to the GPwSI

Having a 'special interest' is nothing new. Traditionally, many GPs over the years have had special interests in subjects such as education, occupational health, management, complimentary medicine and many others. Their role in undergraduate and postgraduate education has not only been recognised but adapted in other fields as well. Take, for example, vocational training in general practice, which is one of the best-evaluated and successful apprentice systems in medicine. Within primary care, some GPs have taken lead roles in their practices for specific clinical areas. These roles have usually centred on general practice tasks, with the exception of minor surgery. In recognition of the fact that if GPs offer minor surgery in primary care it would result in quicker and more convenient service for the patient, an incentive was incorporated into the 1990 GP Contract.[3]

During the period of fundholding, GPs were given incentives for providing services not normally considered as core services to their patients, either by themselves or by commissioning secondary care services. Although this resulted in fragmentation and inequity between fundholders and non-fundholders, it did however act as a catalyst for GPs to acquire further skills not normally considered as a core function of general practice. It was recognised that a significant number of GPs were fully competent to perform a wider range of services than are included within general medical services (GMS), and in order to protect and further patient interests a working group produced guidelines on them.[4]

In 1996, the working group set up by the Department of Health reported that some GPs had skills to carry out a wider range of tasks than were currently included within their contracts. This led to the production of a set of guidelines whereby the health authorities could authorise the provision by GPs of some secondary care services within the primary care setting.[4] Many health authorities approved a few applications, but, in contrast, Bradford Health Authority approved 200 applications and thus became the centre point of research and evaluation with regard to GPwSI.

Fundholding came to an end in 1999 and was replaced by primary care organisations (PCOs), which were initially called primary care groups (PCGs), and later evolved into primary care trusts (PCTS). A cross-sectional survey done in 2001/2002 gave some idea of the numbers of GPs pursuing an outside clinical interest.[5] Although only 40% of the questionnaires sent were adequately completed and returned, more than 70% of the responders indicated that they had at least one special clinical interest and these clinical interests covered over 60 different clinical topics. The vast majority were working as clinical assistants in hospitals, followed by hospital practitioners, with fewer working for the PCG or PCT. In the survey 40% of GPs undertaking special interest work had no contract in place, perhaps undertaking the work in their own practice or privately. The authors of the study concluded that even if none of the non-responders undertook clinical sessions, just by extrapolating the findings of the survey one could assume that there were already 4000 GPs having some special clinical interest outside the realm of traditional general practice. To put it in another way, this would mean that even by very conservative estimates nearly 20% of GPs at the time of this survey had some outside special interest.

Obviously this finding raised the question as to what was new about GPwSI when we have always had GPs with so-called special interests. It perhaps boils down to giving structure and recognition to their training and work. The key pledge of *The NHS Plan*[6] was to establish 1000 specialist GPwSI by 2004'. In April 2002, the Department of Health and the Royal College of General Practitioners (RCGP) published a paper on implementing a scheme for GPwSI. This stated that there may already have been more than 4000 GPwSI at the time and 'many of these posts will continue, but some GPs will wish to enter a scheme which offers an appropriate contract, facilities, support and professional development'. The paper also went on to say that although the term was restricted to GPs, there were many other health professionals, such as nurses, optometrists or dentists, who adopted a similar enhanced role.

The term 'GPwSI' evolved from being called 'specialist GPs' to 'GPs with special interest'. The term is further restricted to mean GPs with special clinical interest rather than any special interest. In the response to *The NHS Plan*[6] the RCGP and the General Practitioners Committee (GPC) of the British Medical Association (BMA) produced their own document,[7] highlighting some of the threats and deficiencies in *The NHS Plan*. They were critical of the term 'specialist GP' as, in their opinion, GPs are all specialists in family medicine, which they thought was a more demanding clinical discipline than most hospital-based disciplines. They were also not in favour of seeing a hierarchical continuum from 'GP' to 'specialist GP' to 'consultant'. They saw each of those roles as equal, but different, in their own way. The response also highlighted the importance of making sure that GPwSIs are not used as a second-class cheap alternative to a consultant service. Although there are generally many advantages, one should not forget the risks associated with having GPwSI.

The NHS Modernisation Agency has published a step-by-step guide to setting up GPwSI services, which includes how to review current service provision, requirements and service design, clinical governance issues, audit and evaluation.[8] The new GP contract[9] encompassed GPwSIs as 'enhanced services' and states that 'these might include more specialised services undertaken by doctors or nurses with special interests' and allowing the PCO to commission whatever they considered appropriate for their locality, thereby setting GPwSIs firmly within the remit of the PCTs.

Advantages and disadvantages

Before analysing the role of the GPwSI, as defined by the Department of Health and the RCGP, we need to look at the threats and opportunities a GPwSI service would provide for GPs, patients, academic institutions and the commissioners of clinical services in primary care.

Implications for the non-specialist

In response to *The NHS Plan*,[6] many universities have started training schemes leading to the award of various diplomas. Notable amongst them was Middlesex University, which offered diploma courses in various subjects, such as ENT and diabetes. The first response from the RCGP was that of caution as the then vice-president of the RCGP warned against the culture of 'diplomatosis', which he feared had the potential to undermine generalist medical practice. He said 'We welcome anything that raises standards for patients, but there is a danger that GPs will feel that if they don't have a diploma in something they won't be able to handle it'.[10] There is therefore a potential for division and conflict within the profession.

Other GPs may be reluctant to refer their patients to fellow GPs who they consider as generalists like themselves. If patients referred to a GPwSI see them in higher esteem than their own GPs or decide to re-register with them it could create further tension within the profession. It is therefore vital that the GPwSI role and its remit is clearly set out at the beginning. Involving the local medical committee (LMC) at the initial stage, along with local GPs within the locality, could avoid these sorts of problems. The other potential source of discontent could come from within the same practice if other GPs are left to compensate for lost time of their colleague, as working one session as a GPwSI is working one session less for traditional general practice. This can only be resolved by having a robust practice agreement and consensus of all within the practice.

There are many advantages as well, such as easy access and more opportunities for feedback both formal and informal. It could also provide better opportunities for educational interaction between GPs and GPwSIs, in contrast to what generally exists between GPs and consultants. A qualitative study looking at the educational interaction between GPs and hospital specialists found a mismatch between what GPs want from specialists in educational terms and what specialists are providing.[11] It also found that specialists preferred traditional, formal teaching methods but GPs preferred informal, problem-oriented learning. It would therefore be logical to assume that a fellow GPwSI would have better understanding of GPs' educational needs.

Implications for GPs working as GPwSIs

With the increasing emphasis on specialisation, even within the same speciality (for example, having a cardiologist with an interest in arrythmias), this is considered as natural progress and general practice could not remain immune to this trend. Interprofessional boundaries are becoming blurred with other allied professionals, such as nurses, taking on the role of what was considered as traditional general practice.

Professionals like doctors and nurses are taking on new tasks and empowering themselves with new skills, so they can offer services both efficiently and cost-effectively. Such extensions of role have provided GPs with intellectual stimulation and an opportunity to further their personal development and heighten their self-esteem.[12] It can also help to prevent them from 'burn out' by giving them job satisfaction and variety. The downside is that they may become victims of inter- and intraprofessional jealousy, leading to isolation and poor morale. It is therefore important and vital to involve all the stakeholders, including the secondary care sector, in the planning as well as the operational stage of the GPwSI service.

Lack of support in the form of manpower as well as the proper facilities needed to run an efficient service can also act as demoralising factors, especially if they are not considered carefully in the planning stage of any new service. One should not forget that the value of generalism might be degraded unless the GPwSI practises within the generalist role. The importance of being a good GP first and foremost is of utmost importance. Lastly, bearing in mind the historical background, there is a need to ensure that GPs are not used as a cheap and second-class substitute for a specialist service.

Implications for patients

The implications for patients are summarised as follows:

- patients' needs are met
- choice: not all patients would prefer to see a GPwSI in place of a consultant,

although a significant majority might

- better access: ease of access is one of the positives that come out of the evaluation of some of the services run by a GPwSI[13]
- shorter waiting times: on evaluating some of the projects especially related to GPwSI-run ENT services, it became obvious that they managed to cut down local waiting lists significantly.[14]

What is not known is the impact of GPwSI on the workload of general practice, also the possible impact on other members of the primary healthcare team and whether it results in longer waiting times to see the GP. There also appear to be gaps in the clinical governance structure in some cases as highlighted by the director of the Department of Health's clinical governance support team.[15]

Cost implications

There is little doubt that cost-effectiveness is one of the factors behind the whole idea of GPwSI, although paradoxically very little is known about it at present. Funding sources for GPwSI are varied and include:

- PCTs
- personal medical services (PMS)
- local development schemes[16]
- earmarked funding for the implementation of particular national service framework
- shifts from secondary to primary care (rarely)
- growth funds.

With various sources of funding, it becomes more difficult to analyse the cost critically. To compound the problem further, economic data may not be as generalisable as clinical studies, and different geographical areas will have their unique local histories, interests and contingencies. Efficiency is not the only criterion that directs health service activity and more important at times is the strength of established interests.

The sessional cost of a GP (at the time of writing) varies between £7000 and £11 000 per year. The paper looking at the economic perspective of GPwSI service concluded:

There is currently no evidence to support these changes from the perspective of effectiveness or cost-effectiveness. In many areas GPwSI development will build on existing historical services that may have actually encouraged inefficient use of resources, e.g. the development of minor surgery in primary care may have encouraged treatment of patients who would not have otherwise been treated and who would have made only a minor impact on hospital workload.[17]

Quite apart from the GPwSI, we need to look at it from an input versus output perspective.

Input (resources)	Output (benefits)
healthcare staff	clinical benefits
medicines	health status and quality of life
premises	non-health benefits, e.g. choice, reassurance, accessibility,
equipment	continuity of care, approachability

Implications for monitoring and evaluation

Few of the GPwSI services have been independently evaluated. Earlier schemes placed little emphasis on formal accountability and monitoring arrangements, relying instead on professional independence and integrity. More formal arrangements are now expected, including distinct clinical and contractual accountability with regular audit and appraisal. Alongside the assurance of high clinical standards and adherence to established protocols, data need to be systematically collected about outcomes for patients.[18] It is therefore essential that all the seven pillars of clinical governance are considered and put in place before embarking upon any GPwSI-run scheme. These are:

- education and training (including ongoing training)
- workload analysis
- health and safety
- staff development
- patient care
- reflective practice
- audit.

In terms of evaluation, we can consider some of the positive and negative reasons for establishing or not establishing a GPwSI service.

Positive reasons

- managing demand
- improving access
- reducing waiting time
- boosting primary care capacity
- to break the monotony of general practice and help prevent 'burn-out'
- to help morale and retention in the workforce
- to compensate for inadequate training at undergraduate and postgraduate levels in certain specialities, such as ENT and dermatology

- reducing inappropriate referrals to secondary care
- improving management of workload between primary and secondary sector
- to help with the education and professional development of GPs.

Negative reasons

- negative impact on already stretched primary care
- may create duplication
- can cause inter- and intraprofessional conflicts
- creates yet another tier of clinical care
- lack of evidence of cost-effectiveness
- lack of proper accreditation in some cases can put both the doctor and patient in a vulnerable position.

To proceed or not to proceed

Whether a GPwSI service becomes an orgy of failure or a shining example of best practice depends as usual on proper assessment prior to setting it up. We have heard the famous saying that 'Good surgeons know how to operate, better surgeons know when to operate but the best surgeons know when not to operate' and the same principle could be applied to setting up any new GPwSI service. To help the PCOs, the Department of Health and the RCGP issued guidelines in 2002, *Implementing a Scheme for General Practitioners with Special Interests.*[19] The Guidelines first identified the priority areas for GPwSI:

- cardiology
- elderly care
- diabetes
- palliative care and cancer
- mental health, including substance abuse
- dermatology
- musculoskeletal medicine
- women, child and sexual health
- ear, nose and throat
- care for homeless, asylum seekers and travellers
- other procedures suitable for community settings (endoscopy, cystoscopy, vasectomies, echocardiography, etc.).

This list is not exhaustive as the PCTs can develop services in other areas if there is an identified compelling local need.

How to proceed

- Identify the area for service development.

- The PCT should look at all the options through its commissioning role.
- If a GPwSI service is identified as the best option then all relevant stakeholders should be involved, including acute trust and staff (consultants, and others), patient groups, local GPs, community and social care services, and local champions, depending upon the area chosen.
- The PCT checks if there are guidelines from the Department of Health and incorporates the framework accordingly. Although there are frameworks in place for most of the priority areas, if for some reason the speciality chosen has no framework, the PCT should contact the Department of Health GPwSI National Development Group (NDG), which will delegate to the RCGP to develop speciality-specific guidelines after consultation with key stakeholders.
- The contract between the GPwSI and the PCT should specify:
  - core activities and competencies required, types of patients suitable for the service, minimum caseload or frequency and reasons for referral*
  - the facilities that must be present to deliver that service
  - the clinical governance, accountability and monitoring arrangements (including links with others working in the same clinical area in primary care) at PCT level and in the acute trust
  - level of payment.

Before the service can be delivered the following must be in place:

- induction, support and CPD arrangements for the GP
- the facilities to allow satisfactory delivery of the service
- the support of the local population, health professionals and health and social care organisations
- local guidelines on the use of the service are widely disseminated
- monitoring and clinical audit arrangements
- appropriate indemnity cover.[18]

Follow-up arrangements

When reviewing the service and the GPwSI work the following should be sought:

---

*Evidence of successful acquisition of the competencies. While an appropriate diploma or similar formal qualification would usually be a credible source of evidence of the acquisition of competencies, many applicants will be able to offer other experience-based evidence. It is important that the service provided meets local needs and that courses and qualifications are appropriate to service requirements. Nationally the Royal College of General Practitioners will advise on the suitability of courses and diplomas for general practitioners with special interests. Locally the postgraduate Dean will be able to give advice.'[18]

- evidence that the guidelines for the use of the service are being followed
- evidence that the caseload is appropriate
- evidence of relevant CPD, clinical audit, exploration of the view of patients, users and other health professionals, peer observation and revalidation
- evidence of involvement in appropriate clinical governance arrangements, including when appropriate in the local acute NHS trust(s)
- evidence of satisfactory process and outcomes of care, including patient views
- evidence that the generalist service is not being adversely affected.

GPwSI role

Although the GPwSI may now be established, the question arises, what are they supposed to do? Three roles have been defined for GPwSI by the Department of Health and the RCGP, as follows.

- To deliver clinical care beyond the normal scope of general practice in the form of either an opinion or clinical service on the request of clinical colleagues (e.g. pigmented lesion clinic).
- To deliver a procedure-based service (e.g. endoscopy and colposcopy, etc.).
- To lead in the development of locality services (e.g. lead in diabetes and cancer, etc.).

The type of role a GPwSI performs depends upon the speciality; for example, a GPwSI in ENT may not necessarily be leading the work in the locality, and someone providing a procedure-based service may not provide expert opinion. Even within the same speciality there may be more than one model in existence as is the case, for example, with ENT.[17]

Skills and training

There appears to be lack of clarity on this issue, as there is no national system for training or accreditation. At present there are two routes for training a GPwSI.

- Experiential: the local committees decide the criteria. It is more locally oriented and GPwSIs going through this route are less mobile.
- Postgraduate diplomas: usually involving one year part-time training with placements for gaining local experience. The downside is the cost implication and it may not be oriented to local needs. GPwSI with recognised qualifications, such as diplomas, tend to be more mobile.

There may also be a mix of both routes.
    As the discussion paper stated:

Some GPs may argue that they have many years experience in dealing with a particular condition and should be allowed to choose the form of continuing medical education that they consider most suitable. Such arguments need to be balanced against the expertise and quality assurance, not least in the eyes of other GPs and patients, that are offered by more formal accreditation[18]

Although it is recommended that the GPwSI supplements the evidence provided by attending a diploma or similar approved course, there is no requirement at present. In which case perhaps the GPwSI should have to gain a set of nationally agreed qualifications to iron out inconsistency and protect patients.

The role of deaneries

The role of deaneries in supporting GPwSI may be summarised as follows.

- In collaboration with the RCGP making the case for GPwSI and defining the attributes of such a practitioner.
- Utilising current deanery education and training programmes or resources to properly support the developing GPwSI role. These might include:
  - higher professional education (HPE)
  - prolonged study leave (PSL)
  - innovative training posts within GP vocational training schemes
  - senior GP registrar posts
  - CPD through appraisal and personal development planning
- Contributing to a regional accreditation panel for GPwSI to create uniformity at local and national levels.

Summary

Although the term 'GPwSI' (still evolving!) is new, the concept is not. However, this new term gives recognition to the training and work of many generalist GPs who have pursued other clinical interests. Like any new initiative there is the danger of going down a slippery path if we lose sight of the original aim and fail to follow the guidelines. GPwSIs are generalists with special interest and not cut-down specialists. As long as they maintain their generalist skills and are trained appropriately for their role, with adequate provisions for their CPD, this can only benefit holistic patient care. It is vital that any intermediate care service utilising a GPwSI is well-resourced and developed in tandem with the PCT (or equivalent body) plans after critically analysing all possible options. There is also the need to have a proper clinical governance framework in place. Overall, the benefits of having GPwSIs outweigh the risks, based upon the available evidence. This evidence is, however, rather patchy and begs further independent research on the subject.

References

1 European Society of General Practice/Family Medicine (2002) *Definition of a General practitioner: consensus statement on behalf of WONCA Europe.* WONCA, Norway.

2 Williams S, Ryan D and Price D (2002) General practitioners with special clinical interest: a model for improving respiratory disease management. *Br J Gen Pract.* **52**: 838–43.

3 Department of Health (1989) *General Practice in the National Health Service.* HMSO, London.

4 Department of Health (1996) *Health Service Guidelines.* HSE (96) 31. DoH, London.

5 Jones R and Bartholomew J (2002) General practitioners with special clinical interests: a cross sectional survey. *Br J Gen Pract.* **52**: 833–4.

6 Department of Health (2000) *The NHS Plan: a plan for investment, a plan for reform.* HMSO, London.

7 Royal College of General Practitioners and General Practitioners Committee of the British Medical Association (2002) *Response to The NHS Plan for England. Intermediate Care and Specialist GPs.* RCGP/BMA, London.

8 NHS Modernisation Agency (2003) *Practitioners with Special Interests. A Step by Step Guide to Setting up a General Practitioner with Special Interest (GPwSI) Service.* NHS Modernisation Agency, London.

9 The NHS Confederation (2003) *New GMS Contract – Investing in General Practice 2003.* Section 2.13. NHS Confederation, London.

10 Royal College of General Practitioners (2001) New round up scheme aims to create 'intermediate' GP specialists. *BMJ.* **322**: 128.

11 Marshall MN (1998) Qualitative study of educational interaction between general practitioners and specialists. *BMJ.* **316**: 442–5.

12 Pringle M (2001) *General Practitioners with Special Interest.* RCGP/RCP, London.

13 Sanderson D (2002) *Evaluation of the GPwSI Pilot Projects within the Action on ENT Programme.* York Health Economics Consortium, University of York.

14 Liu HL (2002) Specialist GPs cut ENT wait. *GP Business.* **18/11**: 40–1.

15 Gerada C (2004) Statement on clinical governance arrangements. *Doctor.* January. p. 3.

16 Primary Care Act 1997. Chapter 46, Section 36.

17 Kernick DP (2003) Developing intermediate care provided by general practitioners with a special interest: the economic perspective. *Br J Gen Pract.* **53**: 553–6.

18 Noon A and Leese B (2004) The role of UK general practitioners with special interests: implications for policy and service delivery. *Br J Gen Pract.* **54**: 50–6.

19 Department of Health and Royal College of General Practitioners (2002) *Implementing a Scheme for General Practitioners with Special Interests.* DoH/RCGP, London.

CHAPTER 21

Clinical ethics and law

John Spicer

Introduction

This chapter begins by reviewing some of the recent trends in clinical ethics education and their relationship to standard ethical analysis methods. Some newer areas of content are then briefly examined and set in the context of this book. The chapter concludes with some suggestions as to the furtherance of study in the clinical law and ethics domain, offering a number of institutions and courses of study that can be undertaken.

Background

To a certain extent this chapter stands out from the others in this book, as it concerns a particular area of potential educational interest, rather than the theory and practice of education in general. There are several reasons for this. First, the study of medical ethics or what we might better call clinical ethics, subsumes all areas of patient care. It is axiomatic that every interaction between a patient and a clinician, even if not face-to-face, has some ethical or legal content.

For the most part that content has traditionally been analysed in terms of dilemmas: moral dilemmas that find medical expression.[1] It is not difficult to identify some of these dilemmas from any area of clinical practice.

- Should this very low birth weight infant, born at 23 weeks' gestation, be treated aggressively?
- Should a clinician discuss a patient's history and management with her relatives and friends?
- Should a doctor acquiesce to a patient's request for a treatment of limited value?
- Should the National Institute of Clinical Excellence (NICE) fund assisted reproduction interventions for all?

Answers to these sorts of questions do not come easily. It seems almost trite to declare, but a number of frameworks for ethical analysis are available to at least attempt resolutions. Perhaps the most popular is the principles framework of Beauchamp and Childress,[2] which can be ruthlessly summarised as follows:

- autonomy: respect individuals' own choices
- beneficence: do good
- non-maleficence: do no harm
- justice: treat equitably.

This framework has been honed over the years[3,4] to the extent that it is the most-quoted ethical analysis for clinical purposes, perhaps even applied overmuch.

Second, the undergraduate approach to clinical ethics education is in transition and advancing fast. In 1998, a seminal paper was published, drawing together departments of medical law and ethics across the UK.[5] A formal syllabus on the subject for medical schools emerged and teaching in this area has expanded enormously. The 12 core themes described by this consensus group were as follows:

- informed consent and refusal of treatment
- clinical relationships: trust, truthfulness and communications
- confidentiality
- medical research
- human reproduction
- the new genetics
- children
- mental disorders and disabilities
- life and death, dying and killing
- vulnerabilities created by the duties of doctors and students
- resource allocation
- rights.

Each of these themes is developed further in the document. The whole represents a core syllabus for the subject and a set of learning aims or goals for all UK medical schools. Those institutions which might seek to curtail it are thus enjoined to explain to their students and quality assurance bodies why that is so. It is fair to say that it will take some time to implement teaching in all these areas, but at least now a road map exists.

Those of us who graduated prior to the implementation of such a syllabus may find ourselves to be relatively undereducated by comparison with our junior colleagues. For this reason, among others, some may seek further learning in law and ethics. This issue is addressed below. It will be noted that the 12 themes contain long-standing issues of clinical ethics, such as confidentiality or life and death, but also newer content. Rights theory, for example, might be termed a relative newcomer to the clinical law and ethics agenda. Given the recent incorporation of the European Convention on Human Rights into UK law, and the utility of a rights-centred morality to argue through clinical dilemmas in clinical practice, this would seem to be apposite. What is not specified by the authors is a teaching and learning methodology, leaving universities to choose their own implementation strategy. The education literature in the last couple of years is full of the various ways in which this is being done, and has many lessons for those of us who work in the postgraduate domain.[6,7,8]

Third and perhaps most interestingly, there is an obvious difference between the study of clinical ethics at a postgraduate level and beforehand.[9] When clinicians have qualified from university they assume patient responsibility almost immediately. They are making decisions on patient care, including diagnosis and treatment. Medicine and allied professions are by their nature vocational. This process offers potential for reflective practice which should be embraced and that should include the ethical and legal aspects of clinical care. Educational supervisors are of course concerned with clinical development, but that offers many opportunities for consideration of the other issues surrounding the clinical. There may be a matter of moral dilemmas, as sketched out above, but may also explore many other areas. Important also, it will be seen, is learning the skills of reflective practice in itself.

A recent additional development is the whole area of ethics support for clinicians. Rather more advanced in secondary care, this concerns support on a case-by-case basis[9,10,11] for clinicians and institutions where ethical issues are identified that need a full discussion and an expert forum.[12] This role is in contrast to the more traditional role of multicentre research ethics committees and local research ethics committees, which are concerned only with research ethical evaluation.

Clinical practice with all its pressures and rewards removes the abstractions often improperly allocated to the study of clinical ethics. Because of this clinicians often seek to study the subject at a postgraduate level, and the opportunities for so doing are described in more detail below.

Some newer ethical challenges

The traditional ethics curriculum has been expanded of late as already described, but the challenges that might be termed 'recent' have a generic pattern that one particular author has neatly identified. This chapter will develop some areas of interest that are rarely covered normally but flow from clinical practice in the early twenty-first century especially in the cities, though certainly elsewhere as well.

Our society has been described as 'increasingly open, litigious and multicultural' and thus 'awareness of the ethical dimension of everything we do is crucial'.[13] Harvey[13] identified, in common with others,[14] *openness* as a positive defining character of not only modern life but also of clinical practice. Accepting that this is so has enormous implications. The word is obviously amenable to differing interpretations but this chapter offers a broad one: when clinicians are open with patients what is described is a relationship uncluttered with unsaid truths.

We might postulate an environment where information of all sorts is available to patients in ways which it might most easily be understood. This might be an account of the information necessary to make a clinical decision autonomously, but also of wider issues. For example, clinicians may have differing roles: as providers of individual healthcare and as commissioners of healthcare. It can be reasonably claimed that where the latter may affect their care, patients should know this. Ultimately, such a rule may lead to a separation of roles in order to avoid conflict of interest. Or another example: often doctors are called upon to write reports on their patients for third parties, such as insurance companies or employers; is that role and responsibility clarified to the patient? To be open is to acknowledge the conflicted role.

Sometimes the conflicted role involves commercial relationships between clinicians as researchers and funding corporations. Recent developments in Canada have led to calls, not just for openness in acknowledging such funding, but even its abolition in the cause of unconflicted knowledge.[15]

These sorts of actions are consistent with recent societal changes anyway and it has been said that healthcare trends reflect social trends. Duncan and Cribb[16] identify three ways in which this can happen.

- Professional authority has been subject to critique from what might be termed 'below': the consumerist. And also from 'above': the influence of encroaching management.
- A greater public understanding of the things that shape our lives.
- Scepticism about professional success criteria so that greater importance is attached to individual decision-making rather than professional.

It could also be said that of the four principles above, respect for autonomy is of greatest importance and merits an ordering above the others. If so, it is sensible to consider openness, honesty and trustworthiness as aspects of clinical practice entirely congruent with respect for patients' autonomous decision-making.

Whether or not our society is more litigious than it was is beyond the scope of this chapter but clinicians' responses to such a threat are undoubtedly within it. Any teacher of clinical law and ethics is aware of the fears of their learners about future negligence claims, in the context of a low professional lifetime risk of law suites. Clinical negligence actions are becoming more common, which seems to evince a greater observed than expected degree of anxiety, so that might afflict individuals. To which it could be added, as do Kennedy and Grub,[17] that the law is an unsatisfactory way of resolving disputes between patients and clinicians.

However, the relationship between law and medicine is complex and a moment's examination may be fruitful. It is necessary to mention again that law is not ethics, and that solutions to the kind of moral dilemmas described above are not usually legal. Furthermore, clinical negligence is but a small part of medical law. What is the greatest part of medical law is that pertaining to specific clinical areas:

- law of consent
- legal issues surrounding death and dying
- the law of confidentiality
- legal issues in reproduction
- mental health law
- clinical negligence.

The law is, of course, always in a state of transition, and at the time of writing there are bills before Parliament concerning human tissue, mental incapacity and euthanasia. The courts hear a constant progression of cases, and negligence claims that have a bearing on interpretation of statute law and thus clinical practice. The Department of Health issues notes and circulars that affect all clinicians and patients and have the status of quasi-law.

Given that clinicians need to be aware of the legal frameworks within which they work, the question needs to be asked as to how this may be kept up to date. For specialists this might be argued to be relatively straightforward, as only rarely do new statutes or important common law affect day-to-day work in a narrow field. For example, pathologists are currently struggling with the implications of the Human Tissue Bill, which emerged after several enquiries.[18,19] Psychiatrists have mounted a lively response to proposals to incarcerate patients with severe dangerous personality disorders on a preemptive basis, part of new mental health legislation.[20] Generalists must be aware of legal issues across a broader field per-haps exemplified by recent Department of Health guidelines on informed consent.[21] Something ostensibly as routine as the seeking of patient's consent to examination and treatment has been re-examined in recent years. This has had a profound impact on clinical practice, in terms of procedure, time and even ethical practice.

When the slightly old-fashioned word 'multiracial' is used in a healthcare context, it is usually a stand-in for 'diversity'. Certainly, there are specific clin-ical and social issues that rise out of considerations of our patients' race, but race is not the only difference between people. We are a diverse collection of indi-viduals in our race, ethnicity, sexual orientation, religion, age, experience and a host of other factors. This is of particular moment in some communities, such as our capital city, rather than other areas which are less diverse.

What must be of importance is that we as professionals learn how to celebrate that diversity and how to best offer care to diverse communities. To take such a position is necessarily moral as well as logical. The ethical arena that seems to be worth examining here is termed 'relativism'. A relativist will accept no universal moral rules, preferring respect for individual groups' moral positions wherever they might be. Whereas the opposite position accords respect to universal moral rules.

This is best illustrated by the UK law on female genital mutilation. This is prohibited, other than for medical purposes.[22] In passing such a law, the UK government accords no respect to tribal customs in Africa, and elsewhere, which include female genital mutilation. Interestingly, that lack of respect does not extend to male genital alteration. A universal moral rule against female genital mutilation is raised into statute law. So for elements of our diverse community that might observe such a practice, the nation is utterly intolerant, for reasons that hardly need rehearsing.

But in other spheres clinicians may have to be relativists, respecting moral rules from within our communities that markedly differ from one another. Dangerous, though, is the possibility of assuming that members of particular communities observe all the cultural norms ascribed to them. One of the side effects of a diverse society is that people mix, and thus do not always maintain the moral norms of their own groups. Respect for autonomy of a personal nature as ever should surely be of prime importance.

There is a professional edge to this as well. As clinicians we are diverse, too; we have origins in the same way as anyone else. Several sorts of question arise here. How might we resolve conflicts between patients and clinicians that might be ascribable to differing moral values based on cultural origin? What are the implications of a manpower crisis that leads us to recruit from other European countries and further afield?

One of the initiatives recently implemented in London was to try and attract doctors from other European nations to help with the manpower shortage currently being experienced. It is not a new phenomenon as, for many years, the UK has needed and benefited from a continuing supply of doctors from all over the world, but it is recently reinvigorated. Such a policy has many implications for deaneries in practical terms, such as achieving successful integration to the NHS, personal development of the clinicians involved and awareness of differing procedures. There are also issues arising from working in a system that may have a different ethical milieu.

As said above, in the UK we have moved from a rather paternalist medical model to one where autonomous decision-making on the part of patients is valued above all. This more subtle aspect of practice is not necessarily valued in the same way in other parts of the world, so therefore a doctor arriving from such a place may need particular guidance and support. Without, of course, undervaluing the medical ethics of their country of origin, it seems that a path between relativism and universal morality must be steered. Whether or not the NHS should be recruiting at all from countries where healthcare professional numbers may be relatively low is also an ethical problem that is rarely addressed.

In addition to all of this, as educators, we are faced with the separate issue of how diversity, relativism and choices can best be taught to a clinical audience. Again, the undergraduate sphere in UK medical education has led the way, detailing a host of different methodologies to advance diversity training.[23] Some work has been reported at a postgraduate level, but it remains an underdeveloped field, ripe for application to all healthcare professionals.

Implications for education

Good education practice requires adequate theorisation: planning learning needs; appropriate teaching and learning methodology; and assessment. Readers may be familiar with the Kolb cycle of experiential learning (Figure 21.1). It is argued that the advancement of clinicians' knowledge, skills or indeed attitudes is best done from the perspective of interactions with patients. In the case of non-clinical specialities, relevant surrogates exist.

It might be further argued that the scope for reflective practice is enormous in clinical ethics. If it is accepted that every patient interaction has ethico-legal content, then every such interaction may merit reflection in this area. Many models for personal reflection exist and whether they are commonly used is arguable, but what should be unarguable is the merit in such a process. Sometimes, such reflection may be guided or facilitated, and indeed it could be said that potentially 'frightening' areas, such as the legal, always need expert input to think through, but this is not necessarily so. For interested clinicians, a wealth of information sources is now available, mainly via the interweb, to complement personal reflection and the acquisition of knowledge.[24,25]

It was argued above that the very fact of professional and life experience rendered clinical ethics a more immediate subject than perhaps earlier in a career. Although the number and quality of many undergraduate assignments gives the lie to such a sweeping statement, nonetheless many clinicians find in their middle careers, a need to study ethics more formally. This could lead to a

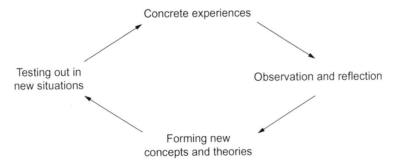

Figure 21.1 The Kolb experiential learning cycle.

structured course at certificate, diploma or masters level. Elsewhere in this book is an account of the mechanics of getting such a course of study approved, implemented and dovetailed with everyday work. What follows is a review of available courses for the pursuance of further interests in clinical ethics and law.

When contemplating such a course the important issues to consider are suggested below:

- uniprofessional or multiprofessional learning group
- part-time or full-time
- transferability of awards
- aims and objectives of each course
- arts-based or science-based
- core content and optional modules
- institutional context
- admission criteria.

Furthermore, careful thought about the following areas is recommended before embarking on such a course:

- aptitude for reading potentially challenging material
- available reading time
- confidence, or willingness, in writing assignments and theses
- willingness to entertain unfamiliar points of view and argue accordingly
- an eclectic approach
- reasoning skills, or the willingness to learn about same
- reflective approach, building on professional experience, but ...
- willingness to set aside professional experience and think objectively.

These suggestions are borne out of the observation of many postgraduate students and reflect, it is hoped, no stereotypical attitudes. It should be said that clinical law and ethics modules are part of many more generalised postgraduate masters courses and the same observations may be made, although to a lesser degree.

In London, courses are available at the following institutions. Space prevents a full comparison between them, so the reader is directed to the referenced websites for further information.

- Centre of Medical Law and Ethics, Kings College:[26] MA in Medical Law and Ethics, MA/PG Diploma in Human Values and Contemporary Global Ethics.
- The Worshipful Society of Apothecaries of London:[27] Diploma in Ethics and Philosophy of Healthcare.
- St Mary's College, Twickenham:[28] MA in Bioethics.
- Imperial College:[29] MSc in Medical Ethics.

Outside London, similar courses are offered all over the UK, including the following.

- Unit for the Study for Health Care Ethics Department of Primary Care University of Liverpool:[30] PG Certificate, Diploma and MSc in Health Care Ethics.
- University of Swansea:[31] PG Certificate, Diploma and MA in Health Care ethics; PG Certificate, Diploma and MA in Health Care Ethics and Law; MA in Medical Humanities.

Increasingly, study can be followed on an extramural basis, via distance learning or even online. Ethics and law in this regard is like any other course, although it should be noted that it is a subject which, if nothing else, is discursive and analytic and thus its study benefits from discussion and shared reasoning. Potential students might also wish to examine the following.

- Manchester School of Law:[32] Postgraduate Diploma/MA in Healthcare Ethics and Law.

There are a number of short courses where healthcare professionals can dip their toes into ethical waters, either to fulfil an interest or decide whether to embark on a full course of study. Notable among them is the following.

- Imperial College:[33] Medical ethics course (five days).

These are a selection of formal taught courses in the clinical ethics domain. It is not necessary to commit to such studying to develop and even relish the subject short of obtaining qualifications in it. Professional journals are rarely without at least review articles on these topics, reflecting its general interest.

Conclusion

It is hoped that readers will take away rekindled interest in the subject of clinical ethics and law, and investigate some of the potential to fan the flames of such a kindling. What can probably not be avoided is the need to have an at least basic knowledge of some of the principles and reasoning discussed above. Indeed, the view might be advanced that mid-career is an ideal time to step slightly back from the mêlée of clinical practice and think more broadly about the care of patients. That thinking may lead into management or education, but also into consideration of ethical themes that have been with us for centuries.

References

1 Battin MP (2003) Bioethics. In: R Frey and CH Wellman (eds) *Companion to Applied Ethics*. Blackwell, Oxford; Chapter 22.

2 Beauchamp T and Childress J (2001) *Principles of Biomedical Ethics* (5e). Cambridge University Press, Cambridge.

3 Gillon R (1987) *Philosophical Medical Ethics*. Wiley, Chichester.

4 General Medical Council (1993) *Tomorrow's Doctors*. GMC, London.

5 Consensus Group of Teachers of Medical Ethics and Law in UK medical schools (1998) Teaching medical ethics and law within medical education: a model for the UK core curriculum. *Journal of Medical Ethics*. **24**: 188–92.

6 Doyal L and Gillon R (1998) Medical ethics and law as a core subject in medical education. *BMJ*. **316**: 1623–4.

7 Goldie J, Schwartz L, McConnachie A *et al.* (2001) Impact of a new course on students potential behaviour on encountering ethical dilemmas. *Medical Education*. **35**: 295–302.

8 Loewy EH (2003) Education practice and bioethics: growing barriers to ethical practice. *Healthcare Analysis*. **11**: 171–9.

9 Goldie J (2000) Review of ethics curricula in undergraduate medical education. *Medical Education*. **34**: 108–19.

10 Slowther A, Bunch C, Woolnough B *et al.* (2001) *Clinical Ethics Support in the UK: a review of the current position and likely development*. Ethox/The Nuffield Trust, London.

11 Slowther A, Johnston C, Goodall J *et al.* (2004) Development of clinical ethics committees. *BMJ*. **328**: 950–2.

12 Peile E (2001) Supporting primary care with ethics education. *BMJ*. **323**: 3–4.

13 Harvey J (2001) Ethics cost, whether you have them or not. *BMJ*. **323**: 336–7.

14 Berwick D, Davidoff F, Hiatt H *et al.* (2001) Refining and implementing the Tavistock principles for everybody in health care. *BMJ*. **323**: 616–20.

15 Shafer A (2004) Biomedical conflicts of interest: a defence of the sequestration thesis. *J Medical Ethics*. **30**: 8–24.

16 Duncan P and Cribb A (2002) *Health Promotion and Professional Ethics*. Blackwell, Oxford.

17 Kennedy I and Grubb A (2000) *Medical Law: text with materials* (3e). Butterworths, London.

18 The Isaacs Report. (www.publications.doh.gov.uk/cmo/isaacsreport/index.htm)

19 The Report of The Royal Liverpool Children's Inquiry. (www.rlcinquiry.org.uk/contents.htm)

20 www.rcpsych.ac.uk/college/parliament/responses/mhbMhlsc.htm.

21 Department of Health (2002) *Reference Guide to Consent for Examination or Treatment*. Department of Health, London.

22 Prohibition of Female Circumcision Act 1985.

23 Dogra N (2001) The development and evaluation of a programme to teach cultural diversity to medical undergraduate students. *Medical Education.* **35**: 232–41.

24 www.bioethics-today.org

25 www.bullmedeth.info/193.htm

26 www.kcl.ac.uk/depsta/law/research/cmle

27 www.apothecaries.org/faculty/index.html

28 www.smuc.ac.uk

29 www.med.ic.ac.uk/divisions/63/msc.asp

30 www.liv.ac.uk/primcare/ethics.htm

31 www.healthscience.swan.ac.uk/Courses/Postgraduate/XMA_Ethics_of_Health_Care.asp

32 http://les.man.ac.uk/law/pg/admissions/mabydl.htm

33 www.ic.ac.uk/cpd/medeth3.htm

CHAPTER 22

The future of postgraduate medical education

Ian Hastie, Neil Jackson and Anne Hastie

Life never stands still as the processes of change continue and the training of doctors is no different. Changes can be seen to affect training in three areas. First, those affecting the trainees or trainers themselves. Second, changes that may occur to the postgraduate medical deaneries and organisations associated with them. Third, changes affecting the medical healthcare system in the UK.

More trainees are wanting to train less than full-time and, although the majority are women, there are a significant number of men who also wish to take up this option. In the past, part-time trainees have usually had super-numerary posts created for them; however, in the future we will see far more opportunities for job-sharing of a training post or the filling of a previous full-time post by a part-time trainee. In addition to this, the European Working Time Directive has brought down trainees' workload to 56 hours per week in 2004 and will reduce it further to 48 hours per week in 2009. Both of these will decrease the availability of training-grade doctors to NHS trusts and they will therefore have to look at alternative ways of providing care to patients. It will also mean that if training continues along traditional lines then a trainee will receive less experience and training within a set timeframe. Consequently, new ways of training doctors, and of allowing them to gain experience, will need to be found.

In 2004, there was an increase in the number of countries belonging to the European Union (EU). Qualifications in one member country are accepted in any other, but we see that in medicine the training in general practice and the medical specialities differs across Europe. In addition to this, the Postgraduate Medical Education and Training Board (PMETB) will be judging the equivalence of training comparable to that of the UK for those doctors who have undertaken training outside the EU. For doctors coming from abroad to continue their train-ing in the UK both these changes mean that proper assessment of their previous training needs to occur in order to be able to fit them into the UK training system at an appropriate point.

Medical training is becoming more competency-based, as opposed to time spent. This will require far more detailed training and assessment for trainees, but also for trainers. It becomes essential to ensure that the principles and purpose of assessment are fully understood given this context. Deaneries have an important part to play in ensuring that a broad range of methods of assessment is used extensively and systematically to determine clinical competence and performance in trainees.

Since postgraduate medical deaneries were established they have continued to develop. The world of medical education in the Nation Health Service (NHS) is complex and dynamic, and our challenge is to manage that complexity today, whilst planning effectively for tomorrow. In recent years we have seen changes to the managerial structure of the NHS and there will be increasing pressures to align the postgraduate medical deaneries with the NHS structure. Deaneries will therefore need to look to their own organisational structures and ensure they are fit for purpose with effective leadership, co-ordinated strategic planning and the effective deployment of resources.

Traditionally, the main links for postgraduate medical deaneries has been to the Department of Health, medical schools or universities and the royal colleges. Other organisations, such as NHS Professionals (which is now a special health authority), workforce development confederations/strategic health authorities and the National Clinical Assessment Authority (NCAA) are now established and links need to be forged between them and the deaneries to enable good working relationships.

The biggest change will be the formation of the PMETB. This will take over the regulation for postgraduate medical training from the Specialist Training Authority (STA) and the Joint Committee for Postgraduate Training in General Practice (JCPTGP). Almost half the members will be non-medical and this will be the first time that a significant proportion of training regulators will be from outside the medical profession. The General Medical Council (GMC) which has itself also undergone a change in membership, will continue to be responsible for undergraduate training, registration of doctors and revalidation of registration.

Healthcare provision continues to modernise and change in the new NHS, where more than 90% of contacts between the population and the NHS take place in the primary care setting. Patients want improved healthcare that is more convenient to them and provided by an appropriately trained workforce. Patients also want, and should be encouraged to take, far more responsibility for their own health. The UK has fewer doctors per head of population than most Western European countries and, although consultant and general practitioner numbers are increasing, it will take several years for an increased number of medical students to be trained to the level that is required for them to give a service to their patients. Some doctors, who have trained abroad or are refugees, can be brought into the workforce but this needs to be done rationally albeit swiftly. In the case of refugee doctors, deaneries have a crucial role in supporting, developing and integrating this valuable resource into the NHS.

Previously, the NHS and private medical services have been separated as far as medical training is concerned. We are now seeing trainees going into hospices run by charitable or voluntary organisations. With the establishment of private treatment centres, which take some of the work from the NHS, we need to place trainees outside the NHS in order for them to become trained in these aspects of care.

Nobody can predict what the future holds, but we do know that change will occur. Education and training support service delivery and we need to make sure that those doctors that we are training will be fit for purpose in whatever healthcare system is operational. Doctors do not just have to be good at diagnosis and treatment but need to be good communicators and good team workers. Some, we hope, will be good trainers.

If deaneries are to be effective in delivering the future of postgraduate medical education they must develop as learning organisations and on this subject, let us leave the last word to Senge.[1]

Learning organisations are possible because, deep down, we are all learners. No one has to teach an infant to learn. In fact, no one has to teach infants anything. They are intrinsically inquisitive, masterful learners, who learn to walk, speak and pretty much run their own households all on their own. Learning organisations are possible because not only is it our nature but we love to learn. Most of us at one time or another have been part of a great team, a group of people who functioned together in an extraordinary way – who trusted one another, who complemented each others' strengths and compensated for each others' limitations, who had common goals that were larger than individual goals, and who produced extraordinary results. What they experienced was a learning organisation. The team that became great didn't start off great – it learned how to produce extraordinary results.

References

1   Senge PM (1992) *The Fifth Discipline – The Art and Practice of the Learning Organisation.* Century Business, London.

Index

Page numbers in italics refer to figures or tables.

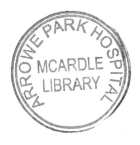